CHAIR YOGA FOR SENIORS

Chair Yoga for Seniors over 60. Transform Your Health: Boost Strength, Mobility and Balance in 28 Days. Lose Weight in 15 Minutes a Day with our Simple Poses

BY MANU LAK

TABLE OF CONTENTS

5   *Exploring the Wonders of Yoga: A Soft Introduction*

8   *The Importance of Gentle and Consistent Exercise for Seniors*

14   *Manifesting Dreams: Goal Setting and Yoga Practice*

17   *Yoga and Psychology: A Relation*

21   *How Does Chair Yoga Lead to Weight Loss*

25   *Cultivating the Right Mindset Before Beginning Daily Practice*

30   *The Importance of Breathing: Exploring Pranayama Exercises*

36   *Embrace Vitality: Essential Exercises for Seniors to Stay Active and Thrive*

71   *Improving Mobility Positions: Tips and Techniques for Seniors*

78   *Muscle Stretching Improvement Positions*

85   *Positions for Improving Balance and Stability*

101   *Day-by-Day Comprehensive Pose Program to Tone, Stabilize and Lose Weight*

108   *Meditation: A Therapy at Home*

113   *Basic Rules of Nutrition during the Practice Month*

Chapter 1

Exploring the Wonders of Yoga: A Soft Introduction

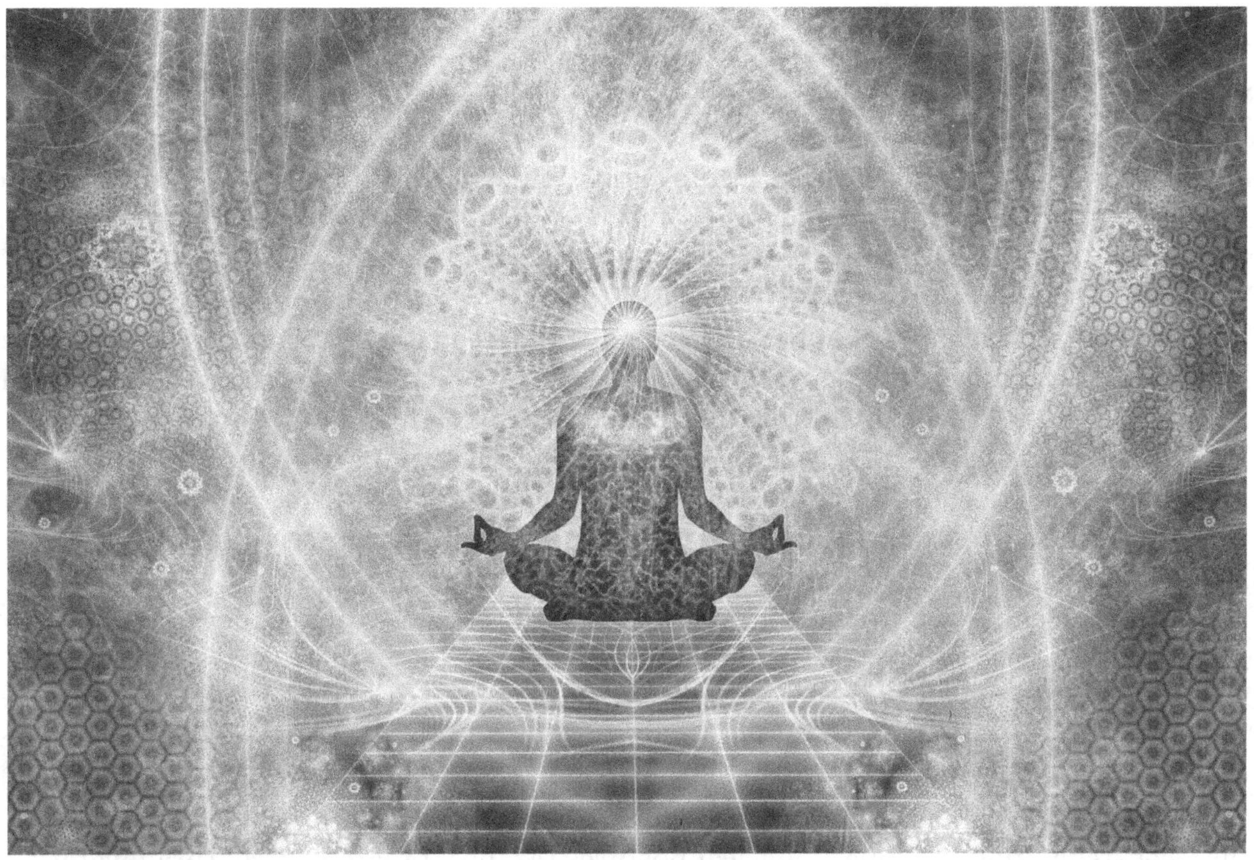

"Yoga is the journey of the self, through the self, to the self."

Welcome, dear friends, to the enchanting world of yoga, where age is but a number and flexibility knows no bounds. Join me as we embark on a delightful journey to unlock the secrets of this ancient practice and rediscover the joy of movement.

What is Yoga?: A Gentle Overview

Yoga isn't just about contorting your body into pretzel-like shapes and losing weight but a way to set your soul free and bring peace to your mind. Yoga fundamentally is a comprehensive approach that integrates the mind, body, and spirit. It's like a magical elixir that brews inner peace, physical strength, and spiritual awakening in a single pot.

Tracing the Threads of Time: Exploring Origins

Let us journey back through the mists of time to the ancient lands of India, where wise sages once sat beneath the whispering leaves of sacred trees, seeking truth and enlightenment. It is here, amidst the timeless wisdom of the Vedas and Upanishads, that the roots of yoga took hold, intertwining with the very fabric of existence.

A Flourishing Tradition: Yoga Through the Ages

Dating back over 5,000 years, yoga emerged from the fertile soil of Indian philosophy and spirituality. Its origins intertwine with the sacred texts known as the Vedas, the earliest scriptures of Hinduism, and the Upanishads, philosophical treatises that delve into the nature of reality and the human soul. These early references to yoga focused on meditation, internal contemplation, and achieving liberation (moksha).

The Indus Valley Civilization and Pre-Vedic Roots

Archaeological evidence suggests that yoga practices might have even predated the written word. Seals and carvings discovered in the Indus Valley Civilization (3300-1300 BCE) depict figures in postures resembling yogic poses, hinting at a possible connection to even older traditions.

The Vedic Period (1500-500 BCE): The Dawn of Yogic Thought

The word "yoga" first appears in the Rig Veda, the oldest Vedic text. Here, yoga refers to a discipline of ritual, sacrifice, and mental discipline. The concept of yoga continued to evolve in the later Vedas, with the emphasis shifting towards self-realization and union with the divine.

The Upanishads (800-300 BCE): Exploring the Inner Landscape

The Upanishads are considered the philosophical heart of Hinduism. These writings explore the essence of the self (Atman) and the ultimate truth (Brahman), presenting yoga as a route to enlightenment.

The Upanishads also discuss the concept of Prana, the vital life force believed to flow through the body's subtle energy channels (nadis).

The Classical Period (500 BCE-800 CE): The Yoga Sutras and the Rise of Schools

This period saw the codification of yoga philosophy and the emergence of distinct schools of yoga. Around 200 BCE, the esteemed scholar Patanjali composed the Yoga Sutras, a seminal text that defines the eightfold path of yoga, known as Ashtanga Yoga. This includes ethical guidelines (yama), self-regulation (niyama), physical postures (asana), breath control (pranayama), withdrawal of the senses (pratyahara), focused concentration (dharana), deep meditation (dhyana), and a state of unity (samadhi).

The Yoga Sutras provided a comprehensive framework for yoga practice, not limited to physical exercises but also incorporating ethical values, mental discipline, and meditative practices. Concurrently, different branches of yoga developed, such as Hatha yoga, which emphasizes physical postures and purification methods, and Raja yoga, which focuses on meditation and achieving elevated states of awareness.

The Post-Classical Era (800-1800 CE): The Development of Tantra and Hatha Yoga

During the post-classical period, Tantra, a sophisticated philosophical and spiritual system, emerged and significantly shaped the evolution of Hatha yoga. Tantric yoga practices placed a greater emphasis on the body's energy channels (nadis) and chakras (energy wheels) and aimed to awaken the dormant kundalini energy at the base of the spine.

The Modern Era (19th Century - Present): Yoga for the Global Citizen

In the 19th and early 20th centuries, yoga began to spread beyond India, introduced by influential figures like Swami Vivekananda. Today, yoga has become a worldwide phenomenon, embraced by millions of people across the globe. While the physical aspects of yoga (asana) have gained immense popularity, many traditions continue to emphasize the practice's holistic approach to well-being, encompassing the mind, body, and spirit.

Now, my dear friends, let us cast aside any notions of age or limitations, for in the world of yoga, anything is possible. Whether you're an experienced yogi or just starting out with your first steps on the mat, there's a spot for you in this wonderful practice.

With each gentle stretch, each mindful breath, we awaken the dormant strength within us, tapping into reservoirs of vitality we never knew existed. As we move through the poses with grace and poise, we begin to feel a sense of lightness, a buoyancy of spirit that carries us through the challenges of life.

So, my dear friends, I invite you to roll out your mats, close your eyes, and breathe deeply, for the journey awaits. Together, let us rediscover the joy of movement, the beauty of stillness, and the boundless potential that lies within each and every one of us. Namaste, dear friends, and may your practice be filled with peace, joy, and endless possibility.

CHAPTER 2
THE IMPORTANCE OF GENTLE AND CONSISTENT EXERCISE FOR SENIORS

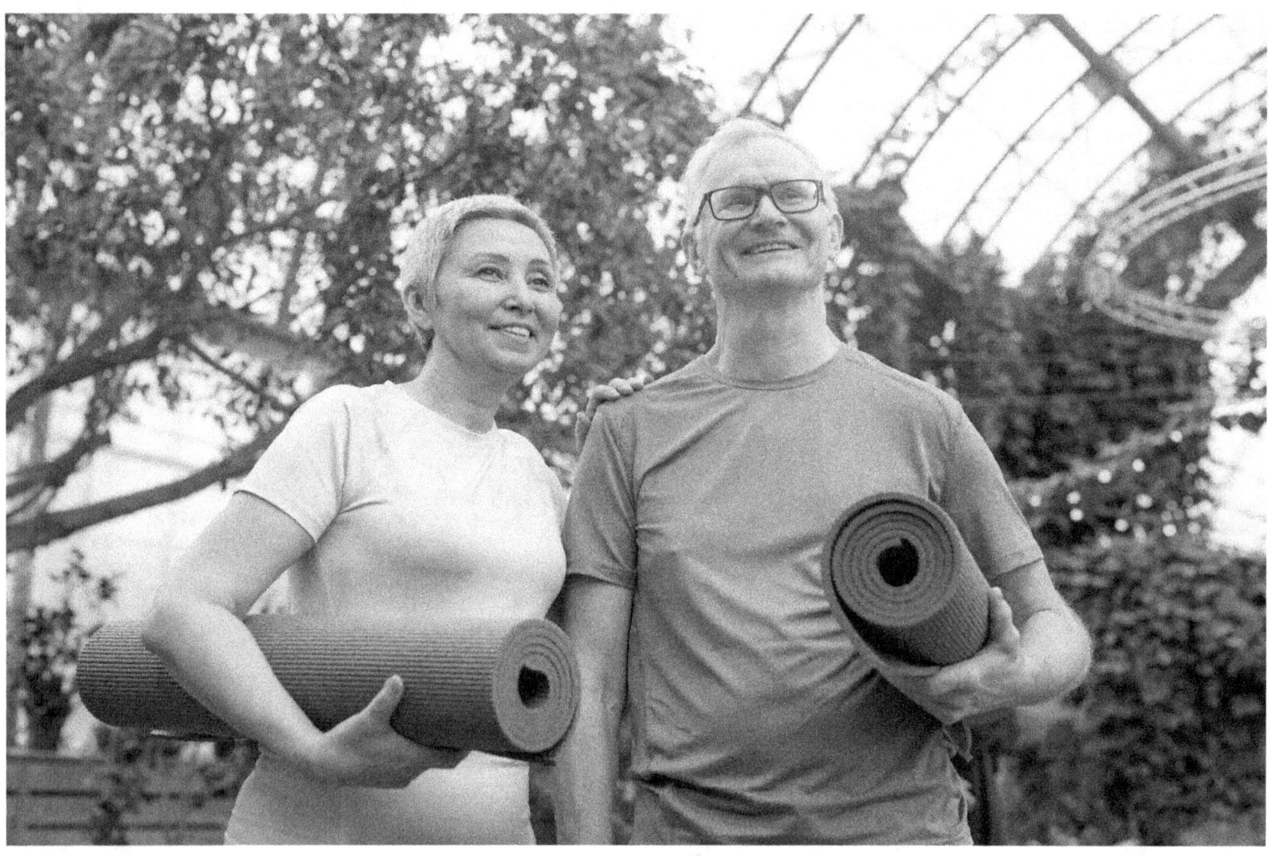

Gentle physical exercise is like a soothing lullaby for the body—a harmonious blend of movements that nurture rather than strain. Picture yourself gracefully gliding through a serene forest, where every step feels like a gentle caress and every stretch a loving embrace.

It's the soft sway of a morning yoga flow, where you gently awaken your muscles and joints with the rising sun. Imagine sinking into a tranquil pool, weightless and free, as the water cradles you in its cool embrace. Gentle exercise is like a gentle breeze that whispers through the trees, guiding you through a series of fluid movements that nourish both body and soul.

Whether it's a leisurely stroll in the park, a refreshing dip in the pool, or a restorative yoga session, gentle exercise is about moving with intention and mindfulness. It's about respecting the needs of your body and discovering joy in the simple act of moving. So, let's embrace the gentle rhythm of exercise and discover the beauty of moving with grace and ease.

Why is regular physical exercise important?

Gentle but consistent physical workouts are not just beneficial but essential for seniors to maintain their health, vitality, and independence as they age. As the body experiences natural changes over time, maintaining physical activity becomes increasingly crucial for overall well-being. Here's why gentle yet regular exercise is crucial for seniors:
- Maintaining Muscle Strength and Joint Flexibility

As we age, our bones undergo a remarkable transformation, and the inevitability of muscle weakening and joint stiffness can pose significant challenges to our daily lives. Simple tasks like reaching for objects on a high shelf or bending down to tie our shoes become increasingly difficult, leading to frustration and a diminished sense of independence.

However, there's hope in the form of gentle exercises that can help mitigate these issues and improve overall quality of life. Activities like walking, swimming, and yoga provide a wide range of benefits for maintaining muscle strength and joint flexibility.

Consider walking, for instance. It's a low-impact activity that can easily be incorporated into daily life. A leisurely walk around the neighborhood not only offers cardiovascular benefits but also activates various muscles across the body, aiding in the preservation of strength and mobility.

Swimming presents a unique chance to work out in a buoyant, low-strain environment, ideal for those looking to reduce joint stress while still achieving a comprehensive workout. The water's resistance enhances muscle strength, and the smooth, flowing movements foster joint flexibility and range of motion.

Yoga, celebrated for centuries for its holistic benefits, integrates mind, body, and spirit. Through gentle stretches and controlled breathing, yoga promotes tension release, better posture, and increased flexibility. Poses like the downward dog, child's pose, and cat-cow stretch target key muscle groups and promote joint health, making everyday movements easier and more comfortable.

- Supporting Bone Health

As we journey through the stages of life, with age comes the risk of *osteoporosis*, a silent but serious condition that weakens bones and increases the susceptibility to fractures. This is particularly prevalent among seniors, especially women, whose bones may become more fragile due to hormonal changes associated with menopause.

Osteoporosis, often dubbed the "silent disease," stealthily progresses without any noticeable symptoms until a fracture occurs, frequently impacting the hip, spine, and wrist with severe consequences such as chronic pain, loss of mobility, and potential disability.

Fortunately, weight-bearing exercises serve as a formidable ally in combatting osteoporosis. These exercises, which involve working against gravity while standing or moving, are proven to stimulate bone growth and enhance bone density, thereby mitigating the risk of fractures and complications associated with osteoporosis.

Walking is a straightforward and effective weight-bearing exercise that can be seamlessly integrated into daily routines. Each step taken while walking supports the body's weight, promoting the deposition of mineral salts like calcium and phosphorus, which are crucial for bone strength and density.

Dancing offers a joyous and engaging method to bolster bone health. Activities such as salsa, ballroom, or line dancing involve rhythmic movements and weight shifts that stimulate bone remodeling and boost bone density. Additionally, dancing is a social activity that enhances mental well-being and fosters social connections, contributing to overall health and vitality.

For those seeking to incorporate resistance into their exercise routines, gentle strength training is highly beneficial. Utilizing light weights or resistance bands, seniors can perform exercises targeting major muscle groups, including the legs, hips, back, and arms. These activities not only build muscle strength and improve balance but also apply forces on the bones to promote growth and density.

While weight-bearing and resistance exercises are pivotal for bone health, they should be complemented by activities that enhance flexibility, balance, and coordination. Yoga, for instance, combines gentle stretches with mindful breathing to improve flexibility and foster relaxation.

Balance exercises like Tai Chi or Pilates are also crucial, as they enhance stability and coordination, reducing the risk of falls and fractures.

Incorporating a variety of weight-bearing exercises into one's routine is key to maintaining optimal bone health as we age. By engaging in activities like walking, dancing, and gentle strength training, seniors can strengthen their bones, reduce the risk of fractures, and enjoy a greater sense of independence and well-being.

- Enhancing Cardiovascular Health

Every little step brings joy to your heart and strengthens it, too. Moreover, uncomplicated activities can do wonders for your heart health.

Imagine yourself in a peaceful garden, tending to plants, or in a park doing slow, graceful movements called tai chi. Tai chi is like a gentle dance that's good for your body and mind. It helps you relax and feel better.

When you do these activities regularly, like taking a slow bike ride, they help your heart in amazing ways. They can keep your blood pressure from getting too high, make sure your blood flows smoothly through your body, and lower the chances of heart problems or strokes.

- Managing Weight and Metabolism

As we age, our metabolism naturally slows down, making it more challenging to maintain a healthy weight. Gentle exercise is crucial in this context as it helps burn calories, build lean muscle mass, and regulate metabolism, thus preventing weight gain and reducing the risk of obesity-related conditions like diabetes and high cholesterol.

Engaging in regular physical activities, particularly gentle exercises such as walking, swimming, or yoga, not only aids in calorie burning but also improves body composition. Building lean muscle through exercise boosts our metabolic rate, meaning our bodies become more efficient at burning calories even when at rest.

Maintaining a healthy weight through exercise lessens the burden on our bodies, especially on the cardiovascular system. Excess weight increases the strain on the heart and blood vessels, heightening the risk of high blood pressure, heart disease, and stroke. By shedding excess pounds and enhancing cardiovascular fitness, we significantly lower these risks.

Furthermore, exercise is key in regulating blood sugar levels and improving insulin sensitivity. During physical activity, our muscles utilize glucose for energy, which helps lower blood sugar levels. Consistent exercise over time can enhance insulin sensitivity, allowing our cells to absorb and utilize glucose more effectively. This is crucial for reducing the risk of type 2 diabetes or managing the condition for those already diagnosed.

Additionally, physical activity has a direct impact on cholesterol levels. Exercise not only helps to lower "bad" LDL cholesterol but also boosts "good" HDL cholesterol levels. This balance is essential for maintaining healthy blood lipid profiles and reducing the risk of atherosclerosis (hardening of the arteries), which can lead to heart attacks and strokes.

So, by incorporating gentle exercise into our daily routines and maintaining a healthy weight, we create a protective shield against obesity-related conditions such as diabetes and high cholesterol. Each step taken towards a more active lifestyle is a step towards better health and longevity.

- Boosting Mood and Mental Health

Engaging in physical activity isn't merely about breaking a sweat; it's a gateway to unleashing a multitude of beneficial effects throughout your body and mind. When you engage in movement, your body releases a mix of feel-good chemicals known as endorphins. These natural mood enhancers fill your system, enveloping you in happiness and well-being, akin to a gentle wave of joy that refreshes and revitalizes you.

The advantages of exercise go far beyond the immediate pleasure. Research has demonstrated that regular physical activity serves as a potent counter to stress, anxiety, and even depression, especially among seniors. By making exercise a staple in your daily routine, you're not only caring for your physical health but also nurturing your mental and emotional well-being.

For seniors, in particular, the effects of exercise on mood and mental health are significant. As we age, we often encounter unique challenges that can impact our emotional state. However, staying physically active helps us manage these challenges, fostering a stronger sense of resilience and contentment.

- Supporting Cognitive Function

Physical exercise is also a powerful ally for maintaining cognitive function and supporting brain health, especially as we age. Research has shown that regular physical activity can have profound effects on the brain, helping to enhance memory, sharpen thinking skills, and reduce the risk of cognitive decline and dementia in older adults.

When we exercise, our bodies release chemicals that promote the growth of new brain cells and strengthen the connections between existing ones. This phenomenon, referred to as neuroplasticity, enables the brain to modify and adapt in reaction to stimuli, which in turn enhances cognitive function.

Furthermore, physical activity boosts blood flow to the brain, supplying it with oxygen and nutrients vital for optimal brain health. This enhanced circulation not only facilitates the growth of new brain cells but also aids in clearing away toxins and waste products that can accumulate in the brain, potentially contributing to cognitive decline.

- Promoting Independence and Quality of Life

Imagine waking up each morning feeling empowered and ready to tackle the day ahead with confidence and grace. For seniors, maintaining independence in daily activities like bathing, dressing, and household chores is not just about physical ability—it's about preserving a sense of autonomy and dignity that enriches life's every moment.

Staying active through exercises that focus on strength, flexibility, and overall fitness is the key to sustaining this independence. When seniors prioritize their physical health, they empower themselves to navigate daily tasks with ease and confidence. Simple activities like gentle stretching exercises can improve flexibility, making bending down to tie shoelaces or reaching for items on high shelves more manageable. Strength training exercises, even using light weights or resistance bands, can assist seniors in maintaining the muscle strength necessary to lift objects, carry groceries, or perform household chores independently.

But, the benefits extend beyond physical capability. By maintaining independence in these activities, seniors foster a profound sense of autonomy and self-reliance. Being able to care for oneself and manage daily tasks without relying on others cultivates a deep sense of pride and accomplishment. It reaffirms one's identity as a capable and active member of the community, bolstering confidence and self-esteem.

Furthermore, this autonomy enhances the quality of life by fostering a sense of purpose and fulfillment. Seniors who preserve their independence are more likely to participate in social activities, engage in hobbies, and enjoy meaningful interactions with loved ones, contributing to overall happiness and well-being. This active engagement with life enhances emotional well-being and overall satisfaction, creating a fulfilling and enriching experience in the golden years.

This commitment to self-care not only enables them to continue performing daily activities independently but also elevates their quality of life, ensuring that each day is lived to the fullest with joy and purpose.

Before embarking on a journey of gentle movement, a visit to your doctor is like tuning an instrument – ensuring everything is in perfect harmony for a beautiful performance. This ensures your exercise program complements your existing health, like a melody composed just for you. Your doctor will listen attentively to your health story, much like a conductor attentively listens to each instrument before the orchestra begins. Performing a physical exam is like fine-tuning the instruments, making sure each one is in optimal condition to create a beautiful symphony. With your doctor's thumbs up, you're ready to begin your harmonious exercise routine, like the conductor raising their baton to start the music.

The beauty of gentle exercise is that it can be a harmonious blend of activities you already enjoy. Imagine yourself gracefully gliding through a serene forest, one step at a time. Walking strengthens your heart, improves circulation, and aids in weight management, much like a gentle melody nourishing your entire being. Imagine yourself on a dazzling lake, floating weightless. Swimming is a full-body experience that strengthens muscles, improves flexibility, and promotes relaxation, like a symphony soothing your mind and body.

Flowing movements, when combined with deep breathing and meditation, create a sensation similar to a calming wave washing over you, providing a tranquil and soothing experience. Tai Chi enhances balance, coordination, and flexibility while reducing stress and promoting inner peace, like a harmonious composition, bringing tranquility. Imagine yourself seated comfortably, like a wise musician preparing to play a beautiful piece. Chair yoga improves flexibility, range of motion, and balance, like gentle notes caressing your body. Let the music inspire your movement! Even low-impact dancing can boost your cardiovascular health, enhance coordination, and improve cognitive function. It's a joyful and social way to express yourself, akin to a cheerful tune that lifts your spirits.

Setting achievable goals is essential for maintaining an exercise routine that resonates like a beautiful melody in your life. Here's how to maintain a rhythmic balance: Start with shorter exercise sessions and gradually increase their duration as you gain strength. Focus on maintaining consistency rather than intensity. Strive to exercise regularly, aiming for most days of the week, even if the sessions are brief. Consistency acts like a constant, soothing rhythm that propels the music forward.

Here are some tips to seamlessly integrate exercise into your daily routine. Treat your exercise time like a cherished appointment in your calendar. This creates consistency and makes it less likely you'll miss your exercise session, like an important note in the melody. Exercising with a friend or family member can boost motivation and make exercise more enjoyable like a harmonious duet enriching the music. Choose activities you find intrinsically pleasing. This will make you more likely to stick with your routine in the long term, like a melody that brings a smile to your face.

Here are some additional tips for a fulfilling movement symphony: Proper footwear is essential to prevent injuries and ensure a safe and enjoyable experience, like having the right instruments for a beautiful performance. This prepares your muscles for activity and minimizes the risk of injury, much like tuning your instruments before a performance. Light cardio and gentle stretches are great warm-up options. Cooldown exercises like walking and static stretches help your body return to its resting state and prevent muscle soreness, like a calming coda at the end of a musical piece. Make sure to drink adequate water before, during, and after exercising to keep hydrated and prevent dehydration, akin to keeping your instrument in top condition. Avoid pushing yourself too hard. If you encounter pain, cease the activity and rest. It's okay to modify exercises or take breaks as needed, like adjusting the tempo of the music to avoid straining the melody.

By incorporating these tips and following a doctor-approved exercise plan, seniors can experience the numerous benefits of gentle and consistent exercise and create a beautiful symphony of movement that enhances their overall health and well-being.

What is the best part? There are many various hobbies to do, so you will discover one that you love. Whether it's taking a stroll in the park or doing simple exercises, each little bit helps your heart stay strong and keeps you feeling good. With the power of *easy* exercises, we can take proactive steps to protect and strengthen our bones, ensuring a lifetime of health, vitality, and mobility.

In conclusion, gentle yet consistent physical exercise is vital for seniors to preserve their health, mobility, and independence as they age. By incorporating regular activity into their daily routine, seniors can enjoy a fuller, more vibrant life well into their golden years.

CHAPTER 3
MANIFESTING DREAMS: GOAL SETTING AND YOGA PRACTICE

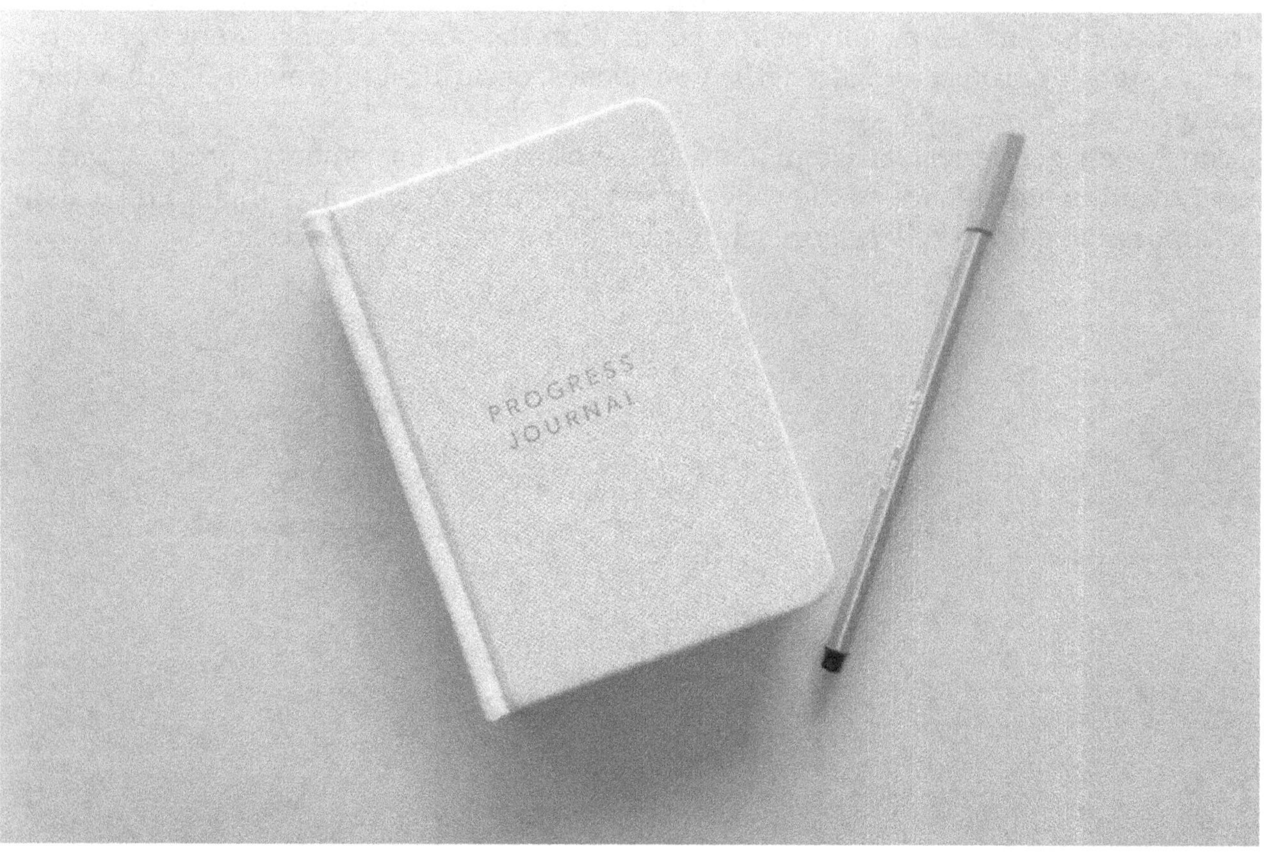

Have you ever felt like you're running in circles, chasing dreams that seem just out of reach? Sarah, a busy professional, felt exactly that way. Juggling work deadlines and personal commitments left her stressed and unsure of how to move forward. Then, she discovered the powerful combination of goal setting and yoga. By setting clear goals and incorporating yoga into her daily routine, Sarah transformed her life.

Imagine waking up each morning feeling energized and focused, clear about your goals and how to achieve them. Picture yourself approaching challenges with a calm mind and a strong body. This is the power of merging goal setting and yoga practice. Both practices work together to cultivate a sense of well-being, clarity, and determination – the perfect recipe for making your dreams a reality.

Goal Setting for Success

Before you embark on your journey of manifesting your dreams through yoga, take a moment to set some goals! This will act as your roadmap to guide you and keep you motivated. According to research, putting your objectives on paper dramatically improves your odds of accomplishing them.

So, bring out a pen and start Setting Your Goals!

Now that your objectives are crystal clear, let's explore this potent technique in more detail.

The journey to manifesting your dreams begins with a roadmap. This roadmap takes the form of clear, actionable goals. People who write down their objectives have a far higher chance of succeeding, according to research. This is the moment to use the **SMART** principle:

- Specific: Clearly and succinctly state your goals. Rather than wishing for "better health," give yourself a specific goal like "running a 5K race within six months."
- Measurable: Create a system for monitoring your development. This may be tracking your training runs and pace for your 5K objective.
- Achievable: Make sure your objectives are tough yet doable. Don't become an overnight marathon runner after becoming a couch potato. Increase your endurance little by bit, starting small.
- Relevant: Ensure that your objectives are in line with your long-term aims and values. Is participating in a5K a first step toward living a better lifestyle, or do you have a stronger affinity for another sport?
- Time-bound: Set due dates for yourself to accomplish each objective. This makes you feel driven and gives you a sense of urgency.

Building Your Routine: Consistency is Key

Remember Sarah? She carved out dedicated time for both yoga and goal reflection in her daily routine. Consistency is essential for success in both areas.

Start small. Set aside 15-20 minutes each day for yoga practice. This could be in the morning to energize yourself or in the evening to unwind. As you progress, you can gradually increase the duration or frequency of your sessions.

Similarly, schedule time for goal reflection. Review your progress, adjust your goals as needed, and stay focused on the big picture.

Yoga offers a wealth of benefits that perfectly complement your goal-setting journey. Here's how:

- Improved Focus and Clarity: Certain yoga poses, like warrior postures or sun salutations, promote mental focus and determination.
- Stress Management: Yoga helps reduce stress hormones, allowing you to approach challenges with a clear head.
- Increased Mindfulness: Yoga teaches you to be present in the moment, enhancing your ability to stay focused on the task at hand.

Weaving the Magic: Combining Practices for Manifesting Dreams

Now, let's talk about creating a space where your goal-setting and yoga practice can flourish. Set up a peaceful space in your house only for these pursuits. Distractions should not be present in this area, and it should be peaceful and calming. It takes effort to remain motivated, remember. Make tiny, attainable objectives for yourself and acknowledge your progress along the way. Setbacks should not depress you; they are an inevitable part of the journey. Treat yourself well and remain dedicated to your path.

Finding Inspiration: Real-Life Success Stories

Sometimes, the best motivation comes from seeing others succeed. Let's take Sarah's story again. By incorporating yoga and goal setting into her routine, she wasn't just running a 5K – she was building a foundation for a healthier and more fulfilling life. Her story exemplifies the power of this approach.

The Science Behind the Synergy

There's more to this dynamic duo than just good vibes. Research shows that both goal setting and yoga have a profound impact on the brain and body. Goal setting activates the prefrontal cortex, which is responsible for decision-making and planning, while yoga reduces stress and improves mood by increasing neurotransmitters like serotonin and dopamine.

Charting Your Course to Manifested Dreams

The synergistic power of goal setting and yoga practice offers a powerful tool for personal growth and transformation. By setting clear goals and incorporating yoga into your daily routine, you can create a life that is aligned with your dreams and aspirations. Start your journey

CHAPTER 4
YOGA AND PSYCHOLOGY: A RELATION

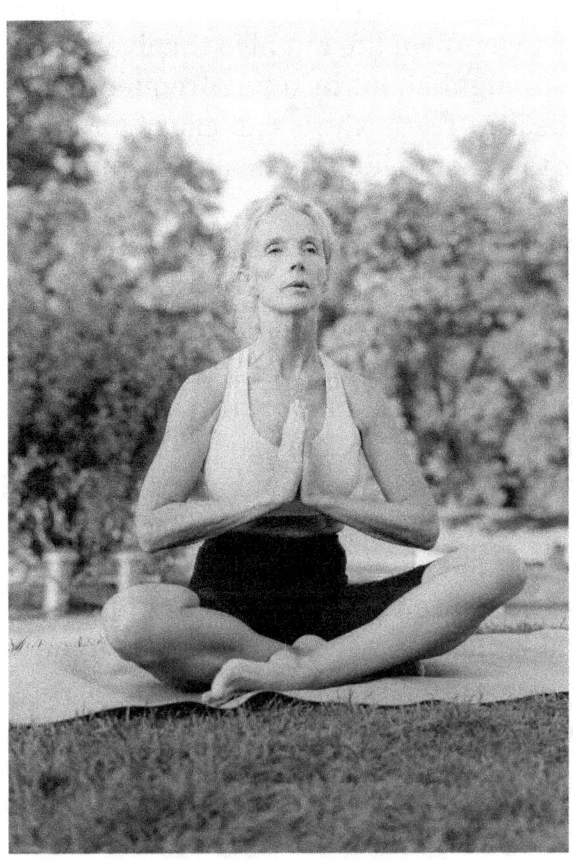

"Age is an opportunity to expand our understanding of ourselves and the world around us."

- Jane Goodall

Have you ever noticed how your memory may not be as sharp as it once was? Fear not, for this is a natural part of the aging process. We'll delve into why these changes occur and how embracing them can lead to a fulfilling senior life.

Welcome, esteemed seniors, to the tranquil oasis of yoga, where each breath is a step towards rejuvenation, and every pose is a testament to your inner strength. As you embark on this journey, imagine yourself stepping into a sacred space where the cares of the world melt away and your spirit finds solace in the gentle embrace of yoga's ancient wisdom.

In this bustling world, where time rushes by like a relentless river, it's easy to feel swept away by the currents of stress and anxiety. The demands of work, family, and the myriad responsibilities that accompany daily life can weigh heavy on our minds and bodies, leaving us feeling drained and depleted. But within the sanctuary of your yoga practice lies a refuge from the chaos—a sanctuary where stress dissipates like morning mist, and the mind finds respite in the stillness of the present moment.

Through gentle stretches, mindful breathing, and guided relaxation, you'll learn to release the tension that binds you, inviting in a deep sense of peace and tranquility that permeates every fiber of your being. With each inhale, you'll draw in calmness and serenity, and with each exhale, you'll let go of worry and tension, surrendering to the gentle rhythm of your breath and the soothing melody of your heart.

Did you know that with age comes a wealth of wisdom? Your happy and difficult life events have molded you into the mature person you are today. Let's honor this insight and investigate how it might improve not just your own life but also the lives of people in your vicinity.

Significant life transitions brought about by aging frequently include retirement, the death of a loved one, or changes in health. These shifts can cause a range of feelings, including anxiety and exhilaration. We'll work together to identify healthy coping strategies so we can handle these transitions with grace and resiliency.

It's normal to reflect on our sense of direction and meaning in life as we become older. Maybe you're looking for new interests to engage in, volunteer work, or community outreach. Let's investigate how finding and pursuing your life's purpose might enhance happiness and contentment during your older years.

Prioritizing our mental health is just as important as prioritizing our physical health. From practicing mindfulness and staying socially engaged to seeking support when needed, we'll uncover practical strategies to nurture your mental health and thrive in your senior years.

But yoga offers more than just physical relaxation—it's a gateway to emotional well-being and spiritual renewal. As you flow gracefully from one pose to the next, you'll feel the weight of the world lift from your shoulders, replaced by a radiant glow of joy and contentment that emanates from within. Your emotional landscape becomes a canvas upon which you paint the colors of happiness and inner peace, each brushstroke a reflection of your profound connection to the present moment and the infinite possibilities it holds.

Psychological Benefits of Yoga for Seniors

. Stress Reduction

Imagine stepping onto your yoga mat feeling a calm and peaceful vibe. As you start your practice, following your breath, you feel like all your worries are melting away. Stretching makes you feel good about yourself and helps you de-stress.

Your body begins to relax with mild stretches, releasing all of the tension held in your joints and muscles. Stretching makes you feel lighter and more liberated, as though a weight has been lifted off your shoulders.

You pay attention to your breathing at the same time. Deep, calm breathing promotes even deeper relaxation in your body. You feel renewed as you take each breath in, and you release any tension or anxieties as you exhale. During your practice, you also pick up mindfulness. This entails focusing on the here and now rather than dwelling too much on the past or future. You get a greater sense of calm when you can examine your thoughts without becoming engrossed in them.

You feel as though your body and mind have taken a small vacation after your yoga practice. You're feeling rejuvenated, at ease, and prepared to face any challenge that may arise. It's similar to embracing oneself and telling yourself, "You're doing great; keep it up!"

. Mood Enhancement

There is more to yoga than only bending and stretching. It's like a whole bundle that looks after your emotions and thoughts. Endorphins are joyful chemicals that your body releases when you practice yoga poses and pay attention to your breathing. They have the same uplifting effects as natural mood enhancers.

You may feel a sense of happiness and contentment rising inside you as you practice yoga positions and take deep breaths. Your body seems to be saying, "Hey, I like this!" You might feel more content with yourself and happy after doing yoga. It's similar to hugging oneself deeply from the inside out.

Yoga is a comprehensive exercise that enhances your mental and emotional health in addition to its physical postures. By engaging in yoga sequences and connecting with your breath, your body releases endorphins, commonly known as 'feel-good hormones,' fostering feelings of joy and contentment.

. Mental Clarity

Amidst life's complexities, yoga serves as a tool to sharpen your mental focus. Through mindful movements and meditation, you cultivate clarity and concentration that extend into your daily activities, making it easier to tackle challenges with a clear mind.

Life can get pretty complicated, right? Well, yoga can help you deal with all that craziness. When you do yoga, especially when you focus on moving slowly and paying attention to what you're doing, it's like giving your brain a workout. You become better at concentrating and staying focused.

Just like when you practice yoga and you try to hold a pose, it takes concentration and focus. And when you sit quietly and meditate, it's like training your brain to stay calm and clear, even when things around you are hectic.

The cool thing is this ability to concentrate doesn't just stay on the yoga mat. It spills over into your everyday life. So when you have to deal with a tough problem or a busy day, you're better at staying focused and thinking clearly. It's like having a superpower that helps you handle whatever life throws at you.

. Self-Awareness

Yoga invites you on a journey of self-discovery, fostering a deep connection between your body, mind, and spirit. Through introspective practices, you gain insights into your inner self, uncovering strengths, and embracing vulnerabilities with acceptance and grace.

Yoga is like an invitation to get to know yourself better. It's not just about stretching; it's about connecting with your whole self—your body, mind, and how you feel inside. When you do yoga, you take time to look inward and understand yourself more deeply.

Through yoga, you learn things about yourself you might not have noticed before. You discover what you're good at and what challenges you. It's like shining a light on the different parts of yourself and accepting them, even the parts that might feel vulnerable.

The cool thing is yoga helps you do this in a gentle way. You learn to be okay with who you are, flaws and all. It's like giving yourself a big hug and saying, "You're pretty awesome, just the way you are."

. Resilience

Life has its highs and lows, doesn't it? But with yoga, you learn how to handle the tough stuff better. Instead of letting problems bring you down, yoga teaches you to deal with them in a strong and positive way.

Yoga helps you learn to go with the flow of life. It's like accepting things as they come and not fighting against them. When you do this, you start to feel stronger on the inside. You realize that you can handle whatever comes your way.

After doing yoga, you feel like you've had a boost of energy. It's like you're ready to take on anything that life throws at you. It's a pretty awesome feeling, knowing that you can handle whatever challenges come your way.

They say age is just a number, and that rings true when we embrace a positive mindset. By focusing on gratitude, resilience, and optimism, you can cultivate a brighter outlook on life, no matter what your age. Let's explore how positive thinking can transform your senior journey. Incorporating yoga into your senior years offers a pathway to holistic well-being, providing not only physical benefits but also nurturing your psychological and emotional health.

Lastly, let's cherish the importance of staying connected with others. Whether it's spending time with family, reconnecting with old friends, or making new connections, nurturing meaningful relationships can bring immense joy and fulfillment in your senior age.

CHAPTER 5

HOW DOES CHAIR YOGA LEAD TO WEIGHT LOSS

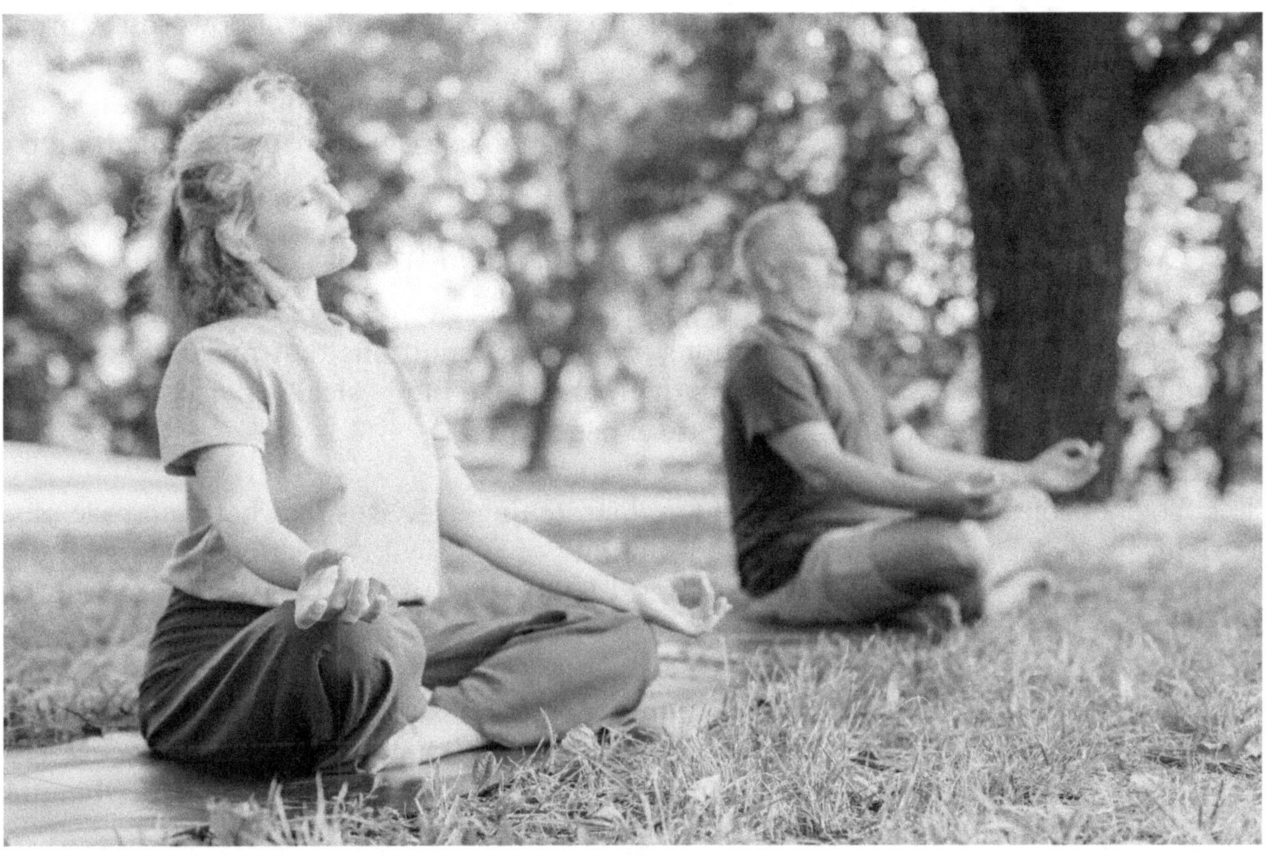

In a world where weight loss is often associated with intense workouts and strict diets. Imagine a form of yoga that allows you to experience all the benefits of a traditional yoga practice while comfortably seated in a chair. Sounds intriguing, doesn't it? Welcome to the world of Chair Yoga – a gentle and accessible way to improve your flexibility, strength, and overall well-being without ever needing to step onto a yoga mat.

What is Chair Yoga?

Chair Yoga is exactly what it sounds like – yoga practiced with the support of a chair. It's a modified form of yoga that adapts traditional poses and breathing techniques to be performed while sitting, standing, or using a chair for support. Designed to cater to people of all ages and physical abilities, Chair Yoga offers a safe and accessible way to experience the physical and mental benefits of yoga.

In Chair Yoga, you'll find a variety of gentle stretches, modified poses, and breathing exercises that can be done while seated comfortably in a chair. These movements are specifically designed to increase flexibility, improve posture, and enhance overall strength, making them suitable for individuals with mobility issues, seniors, office workers, or anyone looking for a more accessible way to practice yoga.

Unlike traditional yoga, where poses may require getting up and down from the floor, Chair Yoga eliminates any barriers to entry by providing a stable and supportive base. This makes it an ideal option for those with limited mobility, chronic pain, or balance issues, allowing them to reap the benefits of yoga without the fear of discomfort or injury.

Moreover, Chair Yoga isn't just about physical exercise; it also incorporates elements of mindfulness and relaxation. Practitioners learn to develop a sense of serenity and inner peace, lowering stress and enhancing emotional well-being via guided breathing exercises and meditation. All from the comfort of a chair, Chair Yoga essentially provides a mild yet powerful approach to enhancing your mental clarity, physical health, and general quality of life. Chair Yoga invites you to experience the transformational power of yoga in a sitting environment, regardless of your goals—recovering from an accident, managing a chronic disease, or just searching for a convenient way to be active.

How and Why Chair Yoga Can Aid in Weight Loss:

Chair Yoga offers a low-impact form of exercise that is gentle on aging joints and muscles. Many seniors may have mobility limitations or chronic conditions that make high-impact activities difficult or risky. Chair Yoga allows them to engage in physical activity safely while still reaping the benefits of movement and calorie expenditure.

- **Increased Physical Activity**

Chair Yoga encourages gentle movement and stretching exercises that help increase physical activity levels, even for those with limited mobility or physical restrictions. By incorporating movements that engage various muscle groups, Chair Yoga can help burn calories and promote weight loss over time.

- **Improved Metabolism**

Regular practice of Chair Yoga can help improve metabolism by increasing blood circulation and stimulating the body's natural processes. The gentle movements and stretching exercises in Chair Yoga help activate muscles and promote better digestion, leading to improved metabolic function and potential weight loss benefits.

- **Stress Reduction**

Chair Yoga combines mindfulness exercises, relaxation methods, and breathing exercises to support emotional and mental well-being and reduce stress. Prolonged stress can cause the hormone cortisol, which is linked to increased hunger and fat storage, to be released, which can lead to weight gain and trouble decreasing weight. Chair Yoga may help people control their weight more effectively and lead healthier lives by lowering stress levels.

- **Mindful Eating**

The mindfulness techniques learned in chair yoga may be applied to other aspects of life, such as eating patterns. Mindful eating can help prevent overeating and encourage healthy food choices. It entails paying attention to hunger indicators, eating carefully, and appreciating every meal. Chair Yoga promotes mindful eating practices, which may help with weight reduction by raising awareness of eating behaviors and dietary choices.

- **Improved Body Awareness**

Chair yoga encourages people to listen to their bodies and respect their physical limits in order to foster better body awareness and self-acceptance. By becoming more attuned to their bodies, individuals may develop a deeper understanding of their hunger and fullness cues, leading to more intuitive eating habits and better weight management.

- **Improved Metabolism**

Regular practice of Chair Yoga can help improve metabolism by increasing blood circulation and stimulating the body's natural processes. The gentle movements and stretching exercises in Chair Yoga help activate muscles and promote better digestion, leading to improved metabolic function and potential weight loss benefits.

- **Increased Energy Levels**

Regular practice of Chair Yoga can help boost energy levels and reduce fatigue, making it easier to engage in physical activity and maintain an active lifestyle. By increasing energy expenditure and promoting a sense of vitality, Chair Yoga may contribute to gradual and sustainable weight loss over time.

- **Targeted Muscle Engagement**

Chair Yoga allows for targeted muscle engagement, making it possible to focus on specific areas of the body, such as the core, arms, and legs. By incorporating targeted exercises and movements, individuals can tone and strengthen muscles in key areas, which may contribute to a more sculpted and toned appearance as part of a weight loss journey.

- **Improved Flexibility**

Chair Yoga includes a variety of stretching exercises that can help improve flexibility and range of motion. Increased flexibility can enhance mobility and reduce the risk of injury during physical activity, allowing individuals to engage in more diverse exercises and activities that support weight loss.

- **Joint Health**

The gentle nature of Chair Yoga makes it suitable for individuals with joint pain or stiffness. By incorporating low-impact movements and stretches, Chair Yoga can help improve joint mobility and reduce discomfort, making it easier for individuals to participate in physical activity and maintain an active lifestyle conducive to weight loss.

- **Mindful Eating**

The mindfulness techniques learned in chair yoga may be applied to other aspects of life, such as eating patterns. Mindful eating can help prevent overeating and encourage healthy food choices. It entails paying attention to hunger indicators, eating carefully, and appreciating every meal. Chair Yoga promotes mindful eating activities that may aid in weight loss by raising awareness of eating behaviors and food choices.

- **Adaptability**

Chair yoga is adaptable to suit the requirements and skill levels of people with a range of physical ailments or disabilities. To ensure that everyone can participate and get the benefits of yoga practice, Chair Yoga includes adaptations and variations for those recuperating from injuries, managing chronic pain, and addressing mobility concerns.

- **Improved Posture**

Chair yoga strengthens the muscles that maintain the spine and body's normal alignment, which can aid with posture. In addition to improving one's looks, proper posture eases the pressure on one's muscles and joints, enabling more comfortable and effective movement when engaging in physical activity.

- **Better Sleep Quality**

Chair Yoga combines mindfulness exercises and relaxation methods to help improve the quality of your sleep. For general health and wellbeing, including managing weight, enough sleep is crucial. Chair Yoga may assist people in getting deeper, more restful sleep by lowering tension and encouraging relaxation, which may aid in weight reduction efforts.

- **Positive Body Image**

Chair yoga encourages self-acceptance and appreciation of one's physical capabilities, which in turn promotes a healthy body image. Regardless of body size or shape, Chair Yoga encourages individuals to focus on what their bodies can do rather than how they look, fostering a sense of empowerment and confidence that supports overall well-being, including weight management.

- **Long-Term Sustainability**

Chair Yoga provides a method for weight control and physical activity that is long-term and sustainable. Unlike more rigorous exercise regimens that may be difficult to sustain, Chair Yoga is gentle, accessible, and enjoyable, making it easier for individuals to incorporate into their daily routine and stick with it over time.

In conclusion, Chair Yoga offers a gentle and accessible approach to weight loss that focuses on holistic well-being and gradual progress. By incorporating gentle movements, stretching exercises, and mindfulness practices, Chair Yoga can aid in weight loss by increasing physical activity, improving metabolism, reducing stress, promoting mindful eating, enhancing body awareness, strengthening core muscles, boosting energy levels, and targeting specific areas of the body.

Whether you're looking to lose weight gradually or simply improve your overall health and well-being, Chair Yoga provides a supportive and sustainable path to achieving your goals.

CHAPTER 6

CULTIVATING THE RIGHT MINDSET BEFORE BEGINNING DAILY PRACTICE

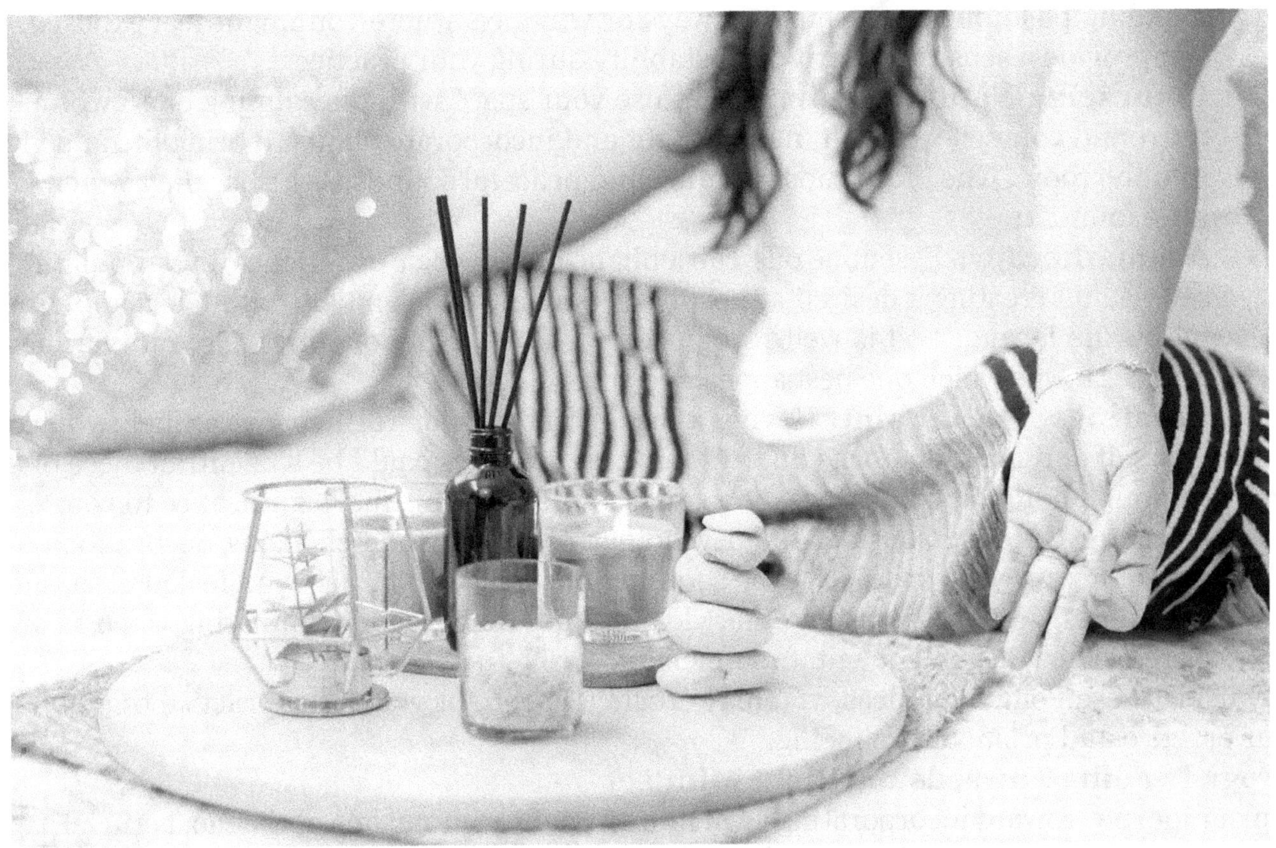

"The mind is everything. What you think you become."

-Buddha

Imagine waking up each morning with a sense of excitement and anticipation, knowing that regardless of what the day may bring, you have the power to shape your own happiness. It's not just wishful thinking; it's the transformative power of the right mindset. By cultivating a positive outlook, embracing gratitude, living with purpose, practicing self-compassion, and fostering resilience, you can unlock the secret to a happier, more fulfilling life. Join me as we explore how a simple shift in mindset can lead to a world of joy and contentment, offering a roadmap to greater happiness and satisfaction in every aspect of your life.

Creating a Sanctuary: Setting the Stage for Your Practice

Before we delve into cultivating the right mindset for your yoga practice, let's consider the environment where this practice will unfold. Your yoga space holds immense potential to influence the quality of your practice. Ideally, it should be a place that fosters tranquility, focus, and a sense of connection with yourself.

Here are some Feng Shui principles you can incorporate to create a yoga sanctuary in your home:

- **Finding the Right Location:** Seek a quiet and clutter-free space in your home. Avoid areas with high traffic or excessive noise. If possible, position your yoga mat in a commanding position, away from doorways or windows where you might feel exposed. This can provide a sense of security and stability during your practice.
- **Embracing Natural Elements:** Infuse your space with the calming energy of nature. Surround yourself with soft, natural light and incorporate plants to bring life and vitality into the room. One of the most calming and peaceful sounds is the trickling water from a little fountain.
- **Aromatherapy:** Essential oils can enhance your yoga experience by stimulating the senses and creating a desired atmosphere. Sandalwood can help with focus and grounding, while lavender oil is well-recognized for its relaxing qualities. Try out various fragrances to see which one best appeals to you.
- **Creating a Focal Point:** Having a focal point in your yoga space can help you center yourself and maintain focus during your practice. This could be a beautiful piece of art, a calming photograph of nature, or a small statue with spiritual significance to you.
- **Inviting Colors:** Consider the psychology of colors when choosing decorations or accents for your yoga space. Choose soothing hues that might help you feel at ease, such as light blues, greens, or whites. Steer clear of hues that are too stimulating, such as orange or red, since they might agitate someone.

By using these Feng Shui ideas, you may create a haven for your yoga practice that enhances your practice and promotes wellbeing.

Yoga Leading Towards the Right Mindset

In our journey toward incorporating yoga into our daily routine, one of the most crucial aspects to consider is our mindset. The attitude we bring to our practice greatly influences not only the physical benefits we gain but also the mental and emotional transformations we experience. Before we dive into the postures and breathing exercises, let's explore how cultivating the right mindset can set the stage for a fulfilling and enriching yoga journey.

A good mindset at the beginning of the day has a ripple effect on the entirety of one's day. A positive mindset in the morning sets the tone for the whole day. It's like planting seeds of positivity that can grow and spread throughout the day.

When we wake up feeling good, it affects everything we do. It makes us more motivated to get things done, and it helps us connect better with others. We also tend to make better decisions and come up with more creative ideas. And when things don't go as planned, a positive mindset helps us bounce back stronger. Overall, starting the day with a positive attitude makes the entire day better.

As seniors, beginning your day ideally involves cultivating a mindset that sets the tone for a fulfilling and rewarding day ahead. Here's how you can approach each morning:

- **Start with gratitude.** Take a moment to appreciate the gift of another day, reflecting on the blessings in your life, be it your health, loved ones, or the simple joys.
- **Set positive intentions.** Think about your goals, your desired emotions, and the mindset you want to project during the day. Having a clear aim can help direct your behavior

and thinking.

- **Practice mindfulness**. Take note of your body's feelings, the flavor of your food, and the ambient noises. Calm and clarity are cultivated by being in the now.
- **Be compassionate with yourself**. Recognize any discomfort or concerns and provide warmth and support without passing judgment. Make your health and well-being a priority.
- **Remain open to possibilities**. Accept the unknown and show yourself open to trying out novel possibilities, viewpoints, and experiences. Remain adaptable and have faith in your capacity to overcome obstacles.
- **Foster connections.** Nurture relationships through conversations, shared activities, or spending time in nature. Building meaningful connections enriches your sense of purpose and fulfillment.

Yoga Leading Towards the Right Mindset

In our journey toward incorporating yoga into our daily routine, one of the most crucial aspects to consider is our mindset. The attitude we bring to our practice greatly influences not only the physical benefits we gain but also the mental and emotional transformations we experience. Before we dive into the postures and breathing exercises, let's explore how cultivating the right mindset can set the stage for a fulfilling and enriching yoga journey.

UNDERSTANDING THE ESSENCE OF YOGA

Yoga is more than just a series of physical movements or stretching exercises. It's a comprehensive approach that includes mind, body, and spirit integration. Fundamentally, yoga aims to balance these aspects, resulting in a condition of vigor, harmony, and inner serenity. As seniors, we have a unique opportunity to embrace yoga as a tool for enhancing our overall well-being, regardless of our age or physical abilities.

Embracing Patience and Self-Compassion

As we embark on our yoga journey, it's essential to cultivate patience and self-compassion within ourselves. It's natural to encounter challenges and limitations, especially as we age. However, rather than becoming discouraged by our perceived shortcomings, let us approach our practice with an open heart and a gentle spirit.

Instead of comparing ourselves to others or fixating on our past abilities, let us celebrate the progress we make each day, no matter how small it may seem. Whether it's finding a sense of ease in a challenging pose or experiencing a moment of stillness in meditation, every step forward is a testament to our dedication and perseverance.

CULTIVATING PRESENT MOMENT AWARENESS

It's simple to let regrets about the past or anxieties about the future carry you away in the fast-paced world of today. But yoga asks us to ground ourselves in the here and now, where genuine happiness and serenity exist. Through practicing mindfulness, or present moment awareness, we may learn to fully appreciate each moment's richness without being distracted by our thoughts.

Let's focus on our breath patterns, the tiny motions of our muscles, and the sensations in our bodies when we practice yoga. We may strengthen our bonds with one another and the environment by remaining mindful of the here and now. This promotes inner peace, clarity, and thankfulness.

Like everything in life, yoga is full of hurdles and disappointments. However, how we handle the difficulties we encounter ultimately decides how successful we are. By maintaining a growth mindset, we can approach difficulties as opportunities for learning, growth, and self-discovery

Instead of viewing limitations as roadblocks, let us see them as invitations to explore new possibilities and adapt our practice to meet our unique needs. Whether it's modifying a pose to accommodate a physical ailment or seeking guidance from a teacher to overcome a mental barrier, every challenge presents an opportunity for growth and transformation.

CULTIVATING GRATITUDE AND JOY

Finally, let us cultivate an attitude of gratitude and joy in our yoga practice. As seniors, we have a wealth of life experience and wisdom to draw upon, and each day is an opportunity to celebrate the gift of being alive.

Whether we're able to fully express a pose or simply find comfort in the gentle movements of our bodies, let us approach our practice with a sense of gratitude for all that it brings into our lives. By embracing the joy of the present moment and savoring the simple pleasures of movement, breath, and stillness, we can infuse our yoga practice with a sense of lightness, vitality, and joy.

As we prepare to embark on our daily yoga practice as seniors, let us remember that the journey begins not with physical postures or breathing exercises but with the right mindset. By embracing patience, self-compassion, present-moment awareness, and a growth mindset, we can lay the foundation for a fulfilling and transformative yoga journey.

With the right mindset, we can unlock the full richness of the yoga experience and discover a renewed sense of vitality, purpose, and joy in our lives.

How to Maintain Healthy Daily Practices

Maintaining healthy daily habits is crucial for boosting general well-being and improving the quality of life for retirees and seniors. A satisfying and lively existence may be achieved by combining mental stimulation, physical activity, a healthy diet, and social interaction. As we age, physical activity is essential to preserving our strength, flexibility, and mobility. Regular exercise that is catered to personal tastes and skills can help fend against chronic illnesses like osteoporosis, diabetes, and heart disease. This might include joint-friendly exercises that are nonetheless very beneficial to health, including yoga, tai chi, strolling, or swimming. Strength training activities can also assist in maintaining bone density and muscle mass, which lowers the risk of fractures and falls. These exercises can be performed with modest weights or resistance bands. Mental stimulation is essential for maintaining mental acuity and cognitive function, in addition to physical activity. Seniors who read, do puzzles, take up new hobbies or talents, and connect with others can all help them keep mental acuity. Engaging in these activities can enhance cognitive function, enhance memory, and focus and perhaps lower the likelihood of dementia and cognitive decline. Maintaining mental activity also promotes a feeling of fulfillment and purpose, which enhances emotional health in general. For seniors, maintaining a balanced diet is another essential component of a healthy lifestyle. Essential nutrients are obtained by eating a range of fruits, vegetables, whole grains, lean meats, and healthy fats. These nutrients maintain optimum health and vigor. Seniors should try to eat foods high in antioxidants for immune system support and disease prevention, omega-3 fatty acids for heart health, and calcium and vitamin D for strong bones. Other crucial practices to sustain energy levels and aid in digestion are eating meals at regular intervals and drinking enough water throughout the day. Participating in social activities is equally vital to older people's general health and wellbeing. Keeping up relationships with friends, family, and neighbors not only lowers feelings of loneliness and isolation but also fosters a sense of purpose and belonging. Depending on their hobbies and interests, seniors might engage in volunteer work, group activities, or join groups or organizations. Additionally, seniors may maintain virtual relationships with loved ones even when they are separated by distance, thanks to technology, which provides possibilities for socialization through online forums, social media, and video conversations. To summarize, maintaining physical, mental, and emotional well-being requires implementing good everyday habits. Seniors may have happy and active lives far into their golden years by placing a high priority on mental and physical stimulation, a healthy diet, and social interaction. These practices not only enhance quality of life but also contribute to longevity and overall happiness.

Chapter 7

The Importance of Breathing: Exploring Pranayama Exercises

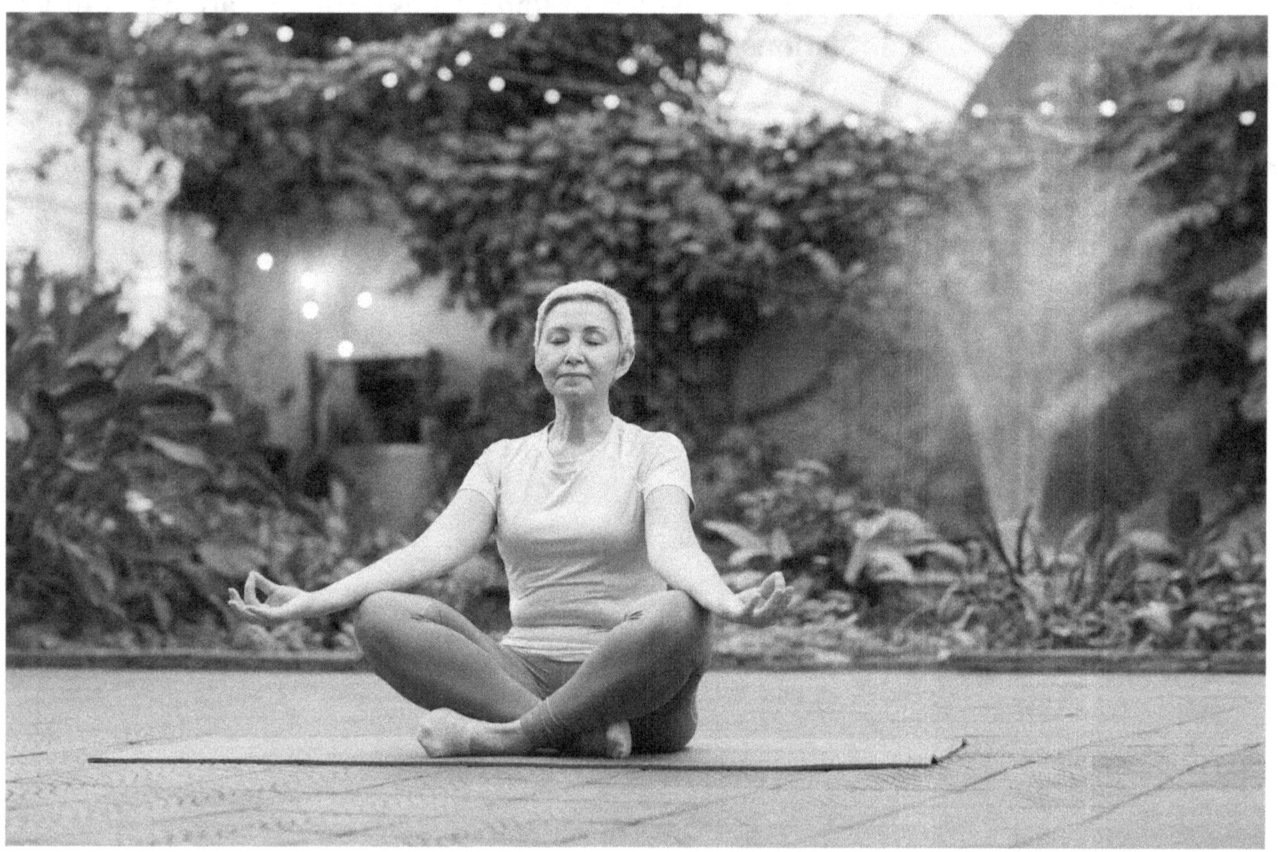

"Inhale the future, exhale the past."

Imagine this: You're standing on your yoga mat, about to start a journey of self-discovery and empowerment. But this isn't just any yoga session—it's an exciting adventure into the mystical world of pranayama, where each breath opens a door to endless possibilities.

As you begin, you feel like an explorer stepping into a dense forest filled with mystery and wonder. Every inhale brings a sense of renewal, like a fresh breeze awakening the senses. And with each exhale, you let go of tension and worries, feeling lighter and more at ease.

Just like exploring the forest, practicing pranayama takes you deeper into yourself. You uncover hidden strengths and insights with every breath, like finding hidden gems along the path. And as you move through each pose, you feel connected to something greater, like tapping into the wisdom of ancient traditions.

In this journey, your breath is your guide, leading you towards inner peace and understanding. With each inhale and exhale, you move closer to your true self, feeling empowered and alive. And as you finish your practice, you carry with you a sense of clarity and strength, ready to face whatever lies ahead.

The Importance of Breath

Breath is the vital link that ties together our physical, mental, and spiritual aspects. When we inhale, we take in crucial oxygen that fuels our cells and organs, while each exhale helps rid our bodies of toxins and tension, promoting relaxation and release. However, in today's fast-paced world, many of us have fallen into shallow, erratic breathing habits, which can lead to stress, anxiety, and a range of physical ailments.

In our modern lives filled with constant busyness and distractions, the natural rhythm of our breath often gets lost. Shallow breathing deprives our bodies of the oxygen they need to function well, causing various health problems. Additionally, shallow breathing keeps our stress response system on high alert, flooding our bodies with stress hormones and contributing to mental and emotional issues like anxiety and depression.

Furthermore, shallow breathing creates physical tension, especially in our neck and shoulder muscles, making it harder to breathe deeply and relax fully. But there's hope. Practices like pranayama (breath control) and mindfulness meditation can help us relearn how to breathe deeply and rhythmically. We can quiet our brains, control our nerve systems, and bring our bodies back into balance by concentrating on our breath. Essentially, we may regain vigor and calm in the middle of life's stress by reestablishing our connection to our breath. It is easy to forget about the basic process of breathing in the everyday rush of life. However, breathing is more than simply a biological process, according to the age-old Pranayama technique; it's a doorway to profound physical, mental, and spiritual well-being. In this exploration, we delve into the importance of breathing according to Pranayama and discover a variety of exercises that can transform our lives.

Understanding Pranayama

Pranayama, often referred to as the science of breath control, is an integral component of yoga practice. In Sanskrit, "prana" means life force or vital energy, while "ayama" means expansion or extension. Together, Pranayama encompasses techniques that regulate the breath to harness and cultivate this vital energy, promoting harmony and balance within the body and mind.

At its core, pranayama serves as a bridge between the body and the mind, facilitating a deeper connection between the two. Through conscious regulation of the breath, practitioners gain mastery over the fluctuations of the mind, leading to enhanced focus, clarity, and emotional stability.

Benefits of Pranayama

Pranayama offers a multitude of benefits for physical, mental, and emotional well-being. By practicing conscious breathing techniques, we can enhance lung capacity, improve respiratory function, and boost immunity. Additionally, Pranayama calms the nervous system, reducing stress levels, promoting relaxation, and fostering a sense of inner peace and tranquility. Moreover, regular Pranayama practice can improve focus, concentration, and mental clarity, leading to greater mindfulness and presence in daily life.

EXERCISE 1: DIAPHRAGMATIC BREATHING

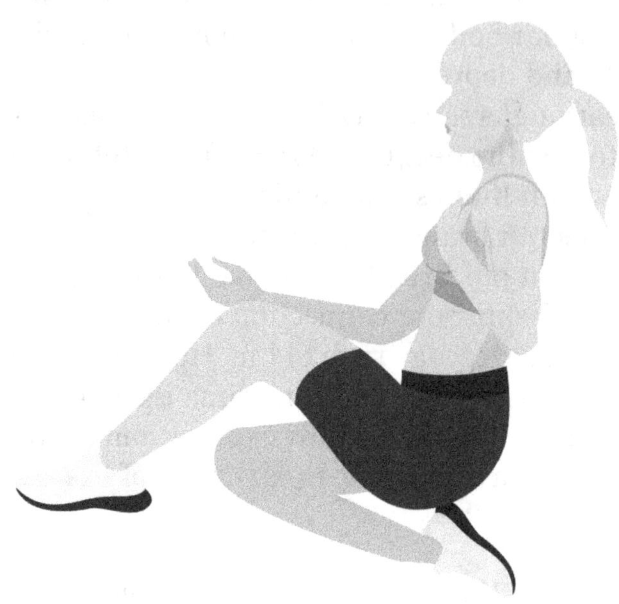

You may learn to breathe more completely and deeply by practicing diaphragmatic breathing, commonly referred to as belly breathing. It's an easy practice that works well. By contracting the diaphragm, the primary breathing muscle, this breathing technique increases oxygen intake and improves breathing efficiency. By focusing on expanding the belly during inhalation and contracting it during exhalation, diaphragmatic breathing can improve respiratory function, increase oxygen flow to the body and brain, and promote a sense of calm and relaxation.

Regularly practicing this technique can also help reduce stress and anxiety by activating the body's natural relaxation response, as well as strengthening the diaphragm muscle itself. Additionally, diaphragmatic breathing can be particularly beneficial for seniors, as it can help counteract the natural decline in respiratory function that often occurs with age, leading to improved overall health and well-being.

Here's how to put it into practice:

- Take a comfortable seat in your chair and space your hip-width apart, feet flat on the ground. Maintain a straight spine and relaxed shoulders.
- Put one hand on your chest and the other, a little below your ribs, on your abdomen.
- Inhale deeply through your nose, paying attention to the expansion of your abdomen throughout the inhale. Under your palm, your belly should lift and expand while your chest stays mostly stationary.
- Let your tummy contract and return to your spine as you gently exhale through your lips. Once more, your chest ought to be mostly still.
- Kbreathing in this manner for five to ten breaths, paying attention to how your tummy rises and falls with each breath in and breath out.

Advice for Breathing Diaphragmatically:
- Try resting on your back with your knees bent and your feet flat on the floor if you first have trouble breathing into your belly. It may be simpler to feel your tummy rise and fall with each breath as a result.
- Spend a few minutes every day practicing diaphragmatic breathing; with time, progressively extend the duration of your practice.
- Keep in mind to breathe deeply and gently, paying attention to how your tummy rises and falls with each breath.

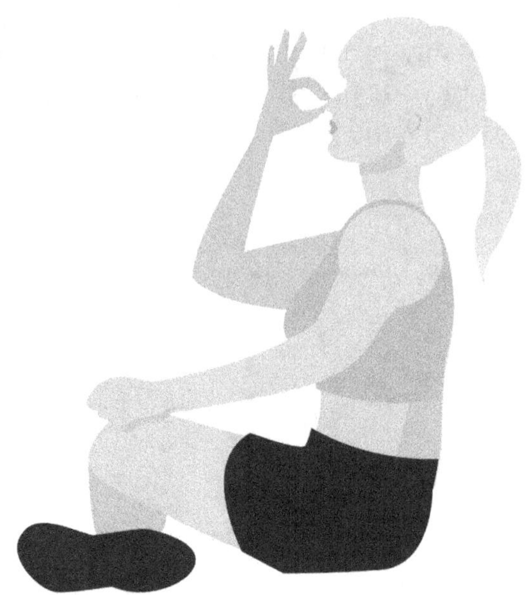

Nadi Shodhana, or alternate nostril breathing, is a potent pranayama method in which one nostril is breathed through at a time in a prescribed rhythm. It is thought that this technique balances the left and right hemispheres of the brain, fostering emotional stability, mental clarity, and attention. This method helps to control the airflow via the nasal passages by switching between the two nostrils, which can enhance respiratory health and boost the body's and the brain's supply of oxygen. By triggering the body's relaxation response, alternate nostril breathing has also been demonstrated to lessen tension and anxiety and to foster a general sense of peace and wellbeing. Regular application of this approach can help elders become more emotionally resilient, increase memory and focus, and improve cognitive performance. Furthermore, by strengthening the respiratory muscles and increasing breathing efficiency, alternate nostril breathing can be a helpful technique for controlling age-related respiratory problems, including shortness of breath or chronic obstructive pulmonary disease (COPD).

Here's how to put it into practice:

1. Take a comfortable seat in your chair, keeping your shoulders loose and your spine straight.
2. Hold your right hand up to your nose and gently shut your right nostril with your right thumb.
3. Breathe deeply via your left nostril until your lungs are completely filled.
4. As you exhale, withdraw your right thumb from your right nostril and use your right index finger to softly seal your left nostril.
5. Gently and fully exhale via your right nostril.
6. Breathe deeply via your right nostril until your lungs are completely filled.
7. Release your right index finger from your left nostril and use your right thumb to softly shut your right nostril at the peak of your inhalation.
8. Breathe out through your left nostril slowly and fully.
9. With this, one cycle of alternating nostril breathing is finished. For five to ten rounds, or

for as long as it is comfortable for you, keep switching between your noses.

Advice on Using a Different Nostril Breath:

- If closing your nose with your fingers is difficult for you at first, try gently pinching it with your thumb and index finger.
- Spend a few minutes every day practicing alternate nostril breathing; with time, progressively extend the duration of your practice.
- Keep in mind to breathe deeply and slowly, paying attention to how the breath enters and exits each nostril.

These two easy pranayama techniques will help you breathe better, feel less stressed and anxious, and cultivate a peaceful, well-being-promoting daily chair yoga practice. It's important to practice frequently and to be kind to yourself while you pick up these new skills. You will eventually start to reap the various advantages of pranayama for yourself with some time and effort.

Incorporating Pranayama into Daily Life

With each breath, you soar higher, delving into the depths of your soul and touching the very essence of existence. Pranayama isn't just a practice—it's an electrifying journey of self-discovery, empowerment, and liberation. So take a deep breath, dear adventurer, and let the magic of pranayama carry you to places beyond your wildest dreams.

Integrating Pranayama into our daily routine can be a transformative practice for overall well-being. Whether practiced as a standalone meditation or integrated into yoga practice, Pranayama offers a simple yet powerful tool for cultivating vitality, resilience, and inner peace. By dedicating just a few minutes each day to conscious breathing, we can tap into the limitless potential of Pranayama to enrich our lives on every level.

The importance of breathing, according to Pranayama, cannot be overstated. By embracing conscious breathing techniques, we can tap into the transformative power of the breath to enhance physical health, mental clarity, and emotional well-being. Through regular practice of Pranayama, we can cultivate harmony and balance within ourselves, fostering a deep sense of vitality, resilience, and inner peace that permeates every aspect of our lives.

By integrating Pranayama into our daily lives, we can infuse each moment with mindfulness and presence, allowing us to navigate life's challenges with grace and ease. Whether it's taking a few deep breaths upon waking up in the morning, practicing Pranayama during a midday break, or winding down with a calming breathing exercise before bed, the opportunities to incorporate conscious breathing are endless.

In essence, Pranayama is not just a series of breathing exercises—it's a holistic approach to life that invites us to embrace each breath as a sacred gift. By honoring the breath as a source of vitality, wisdom, and inner peace, we can unlock the full potential of Pranayama to transform our lives from the inside out.

CHAPTER 8

EMBRACE VITALITY: ESSENTIAL EXERCISES FOR SENIORS TO STAY ACTIVE AND THRIVE

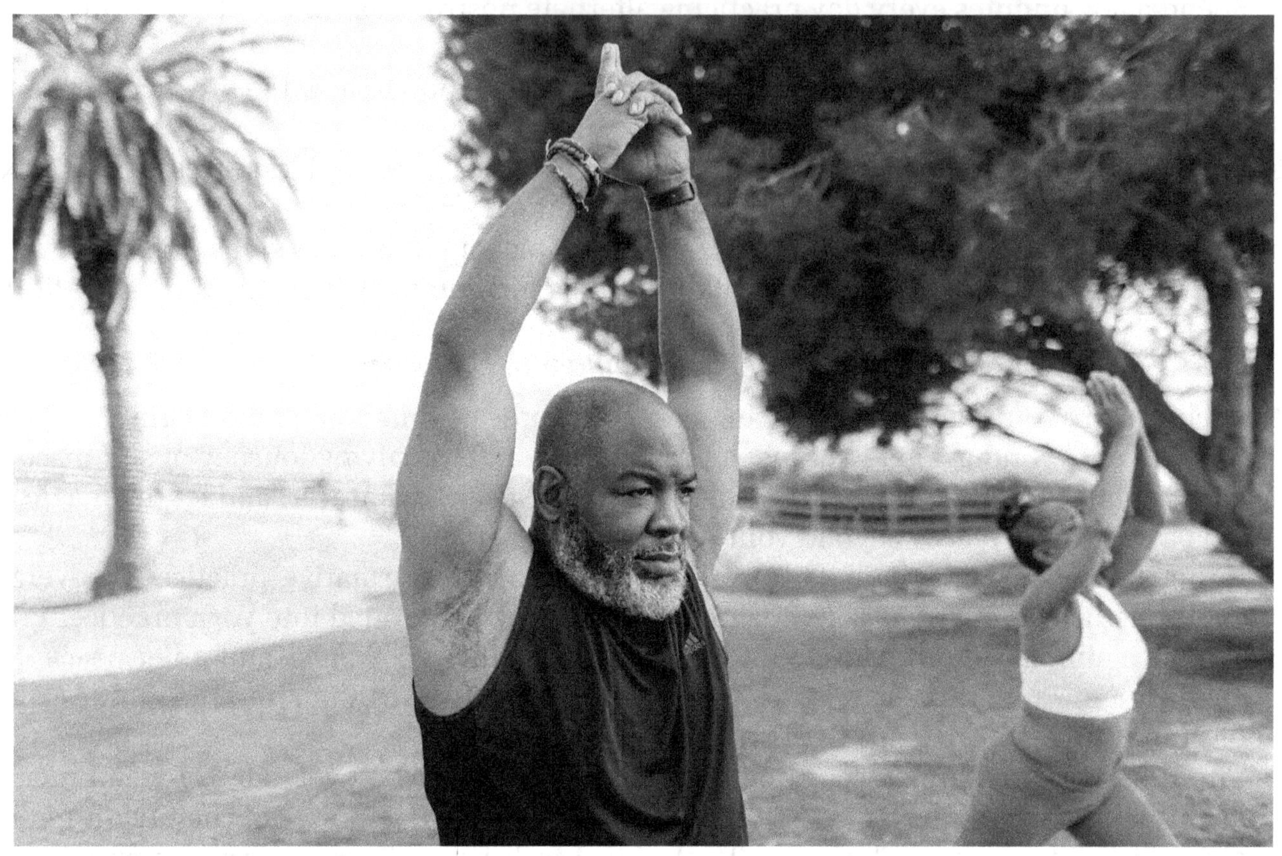

"Exercise is the key not only to physical health but to peace of mind."

- Nelson Mandela

Starting Position

Before beginning any chair yoga practice, it is crucial to find a comfortable and stable seated position that will allow you to perform the exercises safely and effectively. The right starting position can help you maintain proper alignment, reduce the risk of injury, and promote a sense of ease and relaxation throughout your practice.

When selecting a chair for your practice, choose one that is sturdy and stable, with a flat seat and a straight back. Avoid chairs with wheels or rockers, as these can be unstable and increase your risk of falling or losing your balance. Additionally, it's critical to check that the chair height is suitable for you, allowing your knees to be at a 90-degree angle and your feet to rest flat on the ground. After selecting your chair, take a seat with your feet level on the ground and hip-width apart. You can support your feet by placing a folded blanket or pillow below them if they are uncomfortable off the ground. By doing this, you can keep your body in the right posture and avoid putting any tension or discomfort on your lower back or legs. Spend a moment sitting in a tall, erect posture on the chair, with your shoulders relaxed and your spine straight. Picture a thread slowly drawing you upward and stretching your spine, linked to the crown of your head. This will assist you in maintaining proper posture and avoiding any upper back rounding or slouching. Place your hands with your palms facing down on your thighs or the chair's armrests. This will give you a sense of stability and grounding and enable you to use your hands for support during the exercises if necessary.

Take a few deep breaths, in through your nose and out through your mouth, before starting your practice. This practice will assist you in bringing your attention and awareness to your body and breath, allowing you to let go of distractions and anxieties and help you become more present in the moment.

You may become aware of any tightness or stress in your body while you breathe, especially in your lower back, shoulders, and neck. Acknowledge these sensations without judgment, and imagine your breath moving into and softening these areas with each exhalation.

Remember that finding a comfortable and stable starting position is an important part of your chair yoga practice and can help you feel more centered, grounded, and at ease throughout your exercises. Take the time to find a position that feels right for you, and don't hesitate to make any adjustments or modifications as needed to ensure your comfort and safety.

In addition to the physical benefits of finding a good starting position, taking a few moments to settle into your chair and connect with your breath can also have powerful mental and emotional benefits. You may lower tension and anxiety, enhance attention and concentration, and foster a better feeling of general well-being by practicing inner peace and stability as well as bringing your consciousness to the present moment.

Before diving into specific chair yoga poses, it's important to warm up your body and get your muscles and joints moving. Here are a few simple warm-up exercises to try:

EXERCISE 3: CIRCLES TO START WARM UP

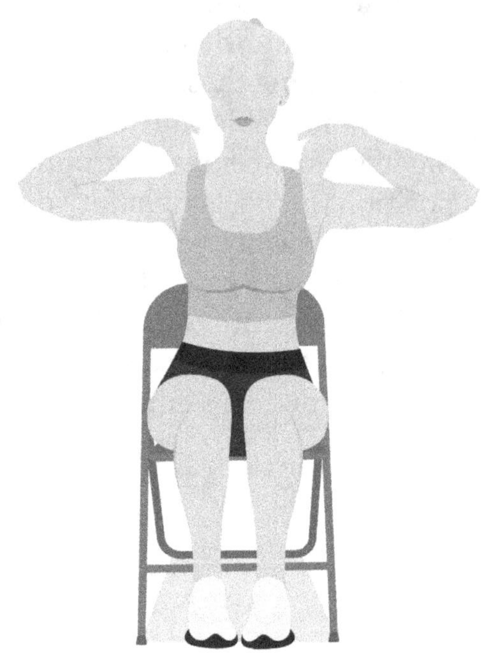

The Circles to Start Warm Up is an excellent way to gently awaken the body and prepare for the rest of your chair yoga practice. This warm-up encourages improved posture and body awareness while also assisting in the augmentation of joint flexibility and range of motion. By moving each joint through its full range of motion, you can help reduce stiffness and tension, leaving you feeling more energized and ready to take on the day.

INSTRUCTIONS:

1. Sit up straight in your chair and put your feet flat on the floor, about hip-width apart.
2. Start by moving your head in small circles, like you're drawing a circle with your nose.
3. Gradually make the circles larger, feeling the stretch in your neck and upper shoulders.
4. After a few circles in one direction, reverse the direction and repeat.
5. Now work on your shoulders. Make small backward and forward circles with your shoulders.
6. Continue the circular motions with your wrists, ankles, and even your torso, moving in both directions.
7. Perform each circular motion for 30 seconds to 1 minute, focusing on your breath and any sensations you feel in your body.

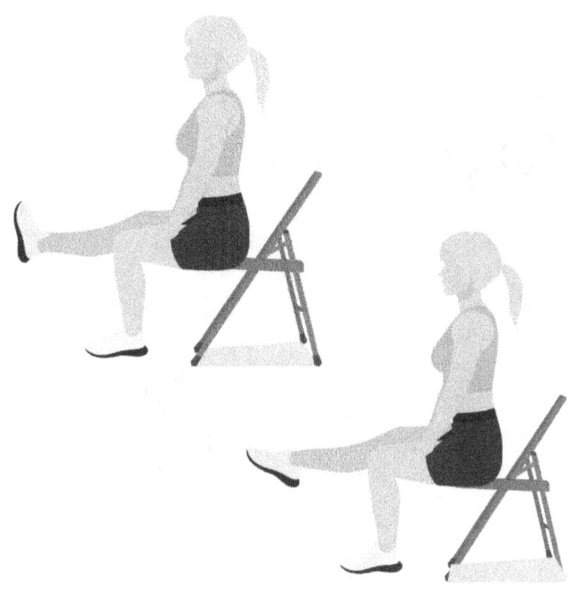

See-Saw Feet Warm Up is a great way to bring some life and energy into your feet and ankles, which can often feel tight and stiff after long periods of sitting. This warmup helps to stretch and strengthen the muscles in the feet and lower legs, while also improving circulation and reducing the risk of blood clots. By challenging your balance and coordination, the See-Saw Feet Warm Up can also help to improve your overall sense of stability and grounding, making it easier to perform other chair yoga poses with ease and confidence.

INSTRUCTIONS:

1. Place your feet flat on the floor, hip-width apart, and sit up straight in your chair.
2. Keep your right leg straight and lift your right foot off the ground.
3. First, point your right toes forward. Then, bend your right foot back toward your shin.
4. Make this see-saw motion continue by bending and straightening your foot back and for-th.
5. If you want to do this for a minute or thirty seconds, switch to your left foot and do it again.
6. To add an extra challenge, try lifting both feet off the ground at the same time and perfor-ming the see-saw motion with both feet simultaneously.

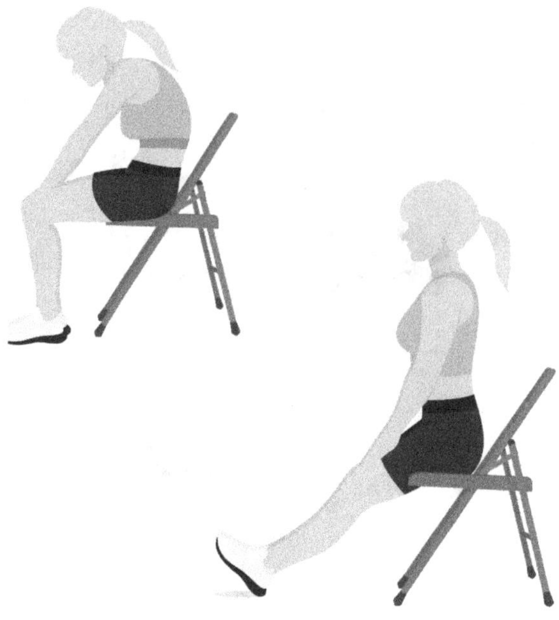

The seated cat-cow stretch is a gentle way to warm up the spine, improve flexibility in the back and neck, and promote good posture and alignment. By alternating between arching the back and rounding the spine, this exercise helps to increase mobility in the back and hips, while also relieving tension and stiffness in the upper body. Regularly practicing seated cat-cow can lead to improved spinal health, reduced risk of back pain and injuries, and a greater sense of overall well-being.

Here are some instructions to follow:

1. Position yourself in a chair so that your feet are flat on the ground and your hands are on your legs.
2. As you breathe in, lift your chest and arch your back. Tilt your head back a little and look up at the ceiling (cow pose).
3. When you let out your breath, round your back, drop your chin to your chest, tuck your tailbone under, and pull your belly button in toward your spine. This is called cat pose.
4. Continue flowing between cow pose on your inhales and cat pose on your exhales for 5-10 breaths, moving slowly and smoothly with your breath.

Tips for Seated Cat-Cow:

- Keep your movements slow and gentle, avoiding any jerky or forceful motions.
- Focus on matching your breath with your action. Breathe in as you arch your back and breathe out as you round your spine.
- If you have any neck or back pain or injuries, move cautiously and avoid any positions that cause discomfort.

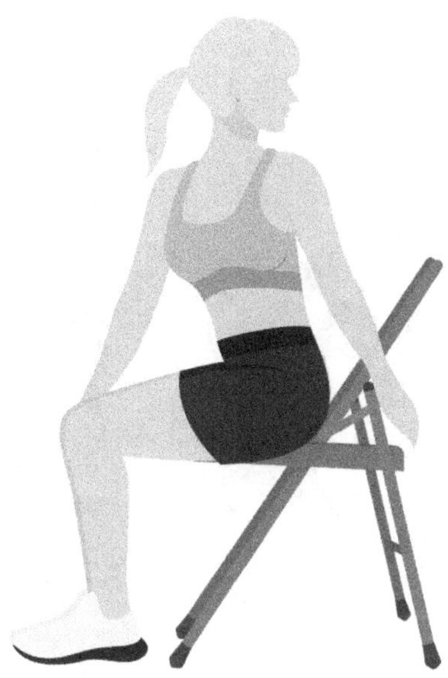

Seated torso twists are a great way to improve flexibility and mobility in the spine, release tension in the back and shoulders, and promote good posture and alignment. By gently twisting the torso to each side, this exercise helps to stimulate digestion, relieve constipation, and increase circulation to the abdominal organs. Regularly practicing seated torso twists can lead to improved spinal health, reduced risk of back pain and injuries, and a greater sense of overall vitality and well-being.

Here are some instructions to follow:

1. Place your feet flat on the floor and your hands on your legs. Sit up straight in your chair.
2. Stretch your back and lift your chest as you breathe in.
3. Keep your hips straight and your feet flat on the floor as you slowly twist your body to the right and let out your breath. You can support yourself by putting your right hand on the outside of your right thigh or on the back of the chair.
4. Focus on stretching your back and taking deep breaths into your belly as you hold the twist for three to five breaths.
5. To release the twist, inhale and gently unwind back to center.
6. Repeat the twist on the left side, twisting to the left as you exhale and holding for 3-5 breaths before releasing back to center.

Tips for Seated Torso Twists:

- Keep your twists gentle and mindful, avoiding any jerky or forceful movements.
- During the twist, focus on making your neck longer and breathing deeply into your belly.
- If you have any back pain or injuries, move cautiously and avoid any positions that cause discomfort.

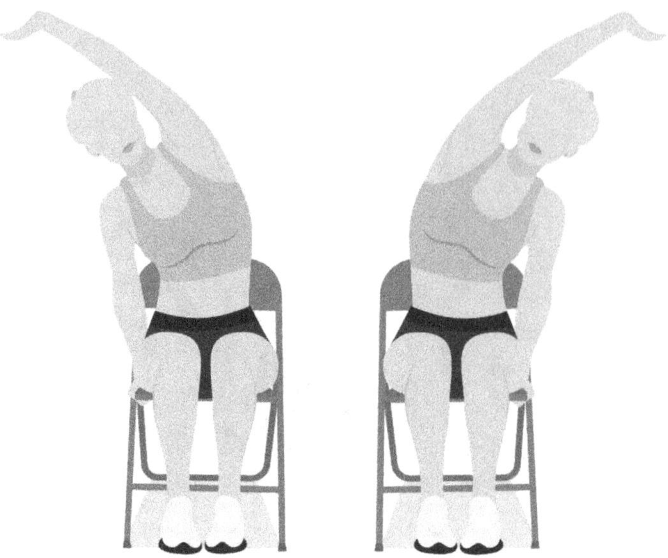

The Lazy Stretch Warm-Up is a great way to loosen up the neck, shoulders, and upper back, which can feel tight and sore after sitting for a long time or having bad posture. This warm-up can help your breathing and circulation by slowly stretching and opening your chest. This can make you feel more energized and refreshed. Aside from that, the Lazy Stretch Warm-Up is a great way to feel more relaxed and calm, which can help lower stress and anxiety and improve your general health.

INSTRUCTIONS:

1. Place your feet flat on the floor, hip-width apart, and sit up straight in your chair.
2. Spread your arms out to the sides and keep them straight out from your body.
3. If you want to slide your shoulder blades into your back pockets, slowly pull them back and down.
4. Inhale deeply through your nose, and then slowly let out your breath through your mouth. This will help your shoulders relax, and your chest open up.
5. As you take your next breath in, reach your right arm up to the sky and then bend slightly to the left. This will stretch the right side of your body.
6. Hold this stretch for three to five breaths, then breathe in and come back to the center.
7. Reach your left arm up and bend to the right to do the stretch again on the other side.
8. Focus on your breath and any body feelings you feel as you keep switching sides for one to two minutes.

The shoulders are a common area of tension and stiffness for many people, especially those who spend a lot of time sitting at a desk or hunched over a computer. Thankfully, chair yoga offers a variety of exercises that can help release tension, improve mobility, and promote better posture in the shoulders. By making these easy but effective moves a part of your daily routine, you can ease upper body pain, lower your risk of injury, and make you feel better overall.

Here are a few chair yoga exercises to help release tension and improve mobility in the shoulders:

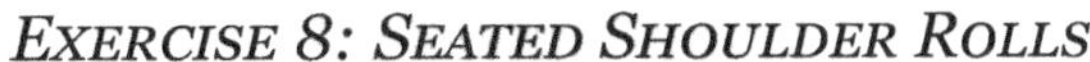

EXERCISE 8: SEATED SHOULDER ROLLS

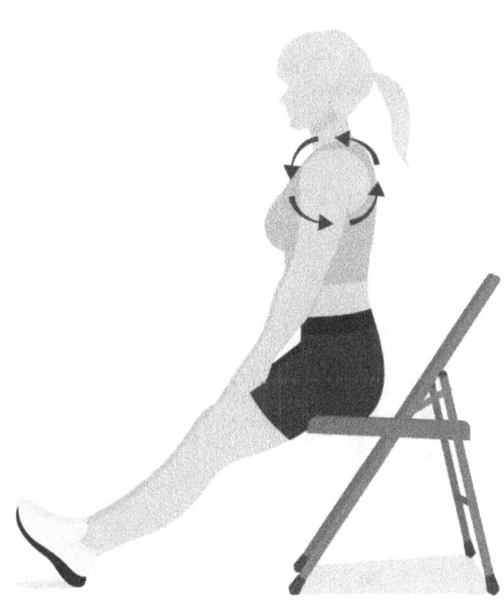

Seated shoulder rolls are a simple and effective way to release tension and stiffness in the shoulders and neck. By gently rolling the shoulders up, back, and down in a circular motion, this exercise helps to improve mobility and range of motion in the upper body while also promoting good posture and alignment. Regularly practicing seated shoulder rolls can help relieve headaches, neck pain, and other common symptoms of tension and stress in the shoulders and neck.

Here are some instructions to follow:

1. Place your feet flat on the floor and your hands on your legs. Sit up straight in your chair.
2. Lift your shoulders up toward your ears as you breathe in. You should feel a stretch in your neck and upper back.
3. When you let your breath out, slowly roll your shoulders back and down. This will bring your shoulder blades together and down your back.
4. Roll your shoulders up, back, and down for 5 to 10 breaths, making sure you move slowly and easily as you breathe.
5. To add a variation, try rolling your shoulders forward on your inhales and backward on your exhales for 5-10 breaths.

Tips for Seated Shoulder Rolls:

- Keep your movements slow and gentle, avoiding any jerky or forceful motions.
- Pay attention to how your movements match up with your breath. Breathe in as you lift your shoulders and out as you roll them back and forth.
- If you have any shoulder pain or injuries, move cautiously and avoid any positions that cause discomfort.

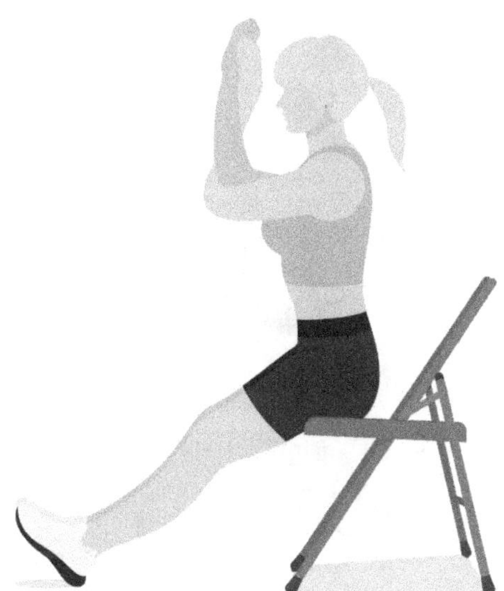

Seated eagle arms, also known as Garudasana arms, are a great way to stretch and open the shoulders, upper back, and arms. By crossing the arms in front of the body and gently pressing the palms together, this exercise helps to release tension and stiffness in the upper body, while also improving posture and alignment. Regularly practicing seated eagle arms can help to promote circulation and lymphatic flow in the arms and hands, leading to greater overall health and well-being.

Here are some instructions to follow:
1. Place your feet flat on the floor and your arms out to the sides at shoulder height. Sit up straight in your chair.
2. Bring your hands together and sweep your right arm under your left arm. Cross your right elbow over your left elbow. Do not put your palms together. Instead, rest the backs of your hands on top of each other.
3. Bring your arms up to your shoulders and lightly press your palms (or the backs of your hands) together.
4. Stay in the pose for three to five breaths, focused on taking deep breaths and letting your shoulders drop away from your ears.
5. To get out of the pose, slowly free your arms and spread them out to the sides again.
6. Repeat the pose on the other side, crossing your left arm under your right arm and holding for 3-5 breaths before releasing.

Tips for Seated Eagle Arms:
- Keep your shoulders relaxed and your elbows lifted throughout the pose.
- If you have any shoulder pain or injuries, move cautiously and avoid any positions that cause discomfort.
- During the pose, focus on taking deep, even breaths. Let your breath help you rest and let go of stress.

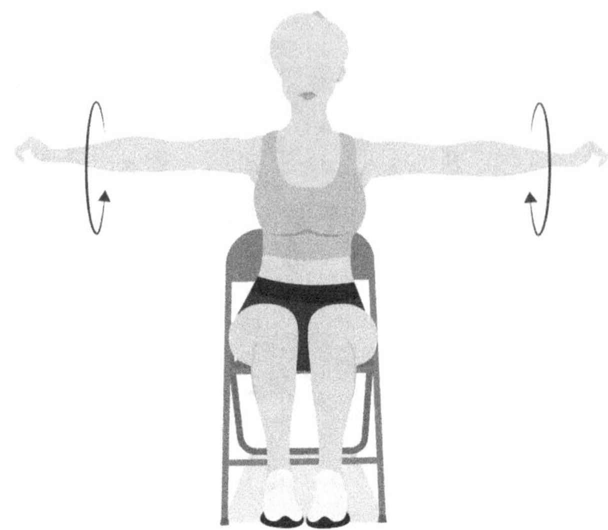

Seated arm circles are a simple yet effective way to improve shoulder mobility and flexibility while also reducing tension in the neck and upper back. By making circular motions with the arms and gradually increasing the size of the circles, this exercise helps to increase blood circulation in the arms and shoulders, leading to greater overall health and well-being.

1. Place your feet flat on the floor, hip-width apart, and sit up straight in your chair.
2. Put your arms out to the sides, shoulder-width apart, hands down.
3. Start moving your arms in small circles, and as you get better, make the circles bigger.
4. 10 circles should go in each direction, and then 10 circles should go the other way.

Tips:
- During the whole practice, keep your back straight and your core tight.
- If the rings hurt or make you feel bad, make them smaller or stop the practice.

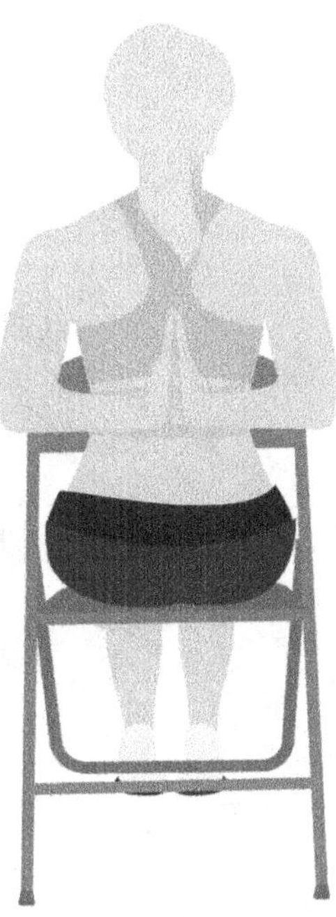

The seated reverse prayer pose is a gentle yet effective way to stretch the shoulders, chest, and upper back while improving posture and counteracting the effects of slouching. By bringing the hands behind the back and interlacing the fingers, this exercise helps to open the chest and relieve tension in the neck and shoulders, leading to greater overall comfort and ease in the upper body.

1. Sit tall in your chair with your feet flat on the floor, hip-width apart.
2. Bring your hands behind your back, interlacing your fingers.
3. If your shoulders are tight, hold a towel or strap between your hands.
4. Straighten your arms and lift your hands away from your back, gently opening your chest.
5. Hold for 3-5 breaths, then release and bring your hands back to your lap.

Tips:

- Keep your core engaged and your spine straight throughout the pose.
- If you feel any strain in your shoulders or wrists, release the pose and try again with a towel or strap.

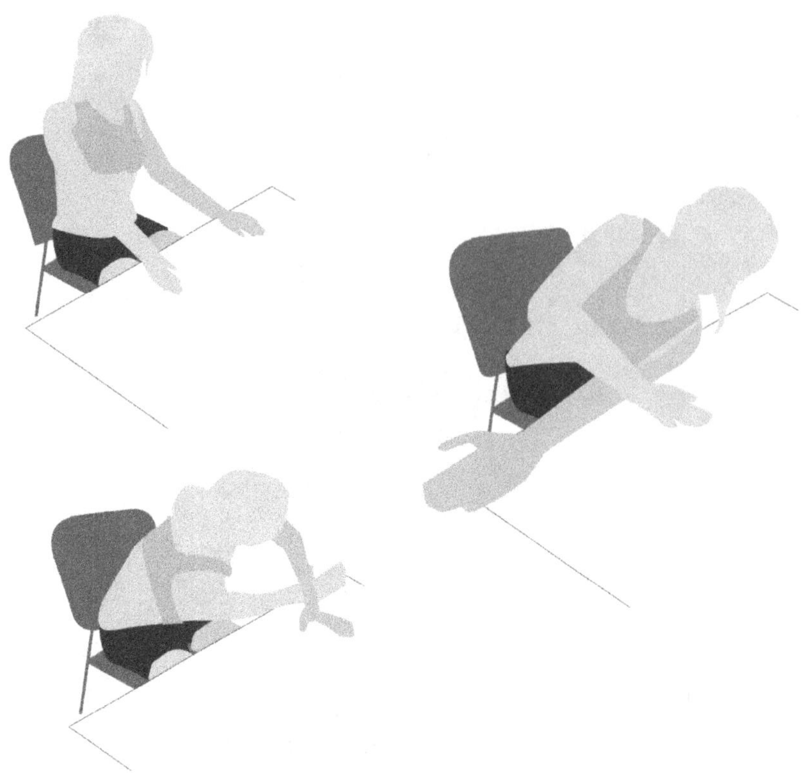

The seated thread of the needle is a gentle yet effective way to stretch the shoulders, upper back, and neck while also improving spinal mobility and flexibility. By raising one arm overhead and threading it behind the opposite ear, this exercise helps to release tension and stiffness in the upper body, leading to greater overall comfort and ease of movement. Regularly practicing the seated thread of the needle can help alleviate common symptoms of tension and stress in the upper body, such as headaches and neck pain.

1. Sit tall in your chair with your feet flat on the floor, hip-width apart.
2. Raise your right arm overhead, then bend your elbow and bring your hand down behind your head.
3. Bring your left hand up to meet your right elbow, gently pressing it downward.
4. Hold for 3-5 breaths, then release and repeat on the opposite side.

Tips:
- Keep your core engaged and your spine straight throughout the pose.
- If you feel any pain or discomfort, reduce the pressure on your elbow or stop the exercise.

The chest is an area of the body that can easily become tight and constricted, especially for those who spend a lot of time sitting or hunched over. When the chest muscles are tight, it can lead to poor posture, shallow breathing, and even neck and shoulder pain. Fortunately, chair yoga offers a variety of exercises that can help to open and stretch the chest, promoting better posture, deeper breathing, and a greater sense of overall well-being.

By incorporating these simple yet effective chest-opening exercises into your daily routine, you can counteract the effects of prolonged sitting and improve your overall upper body mobility and function. These exercises are gentle enough for people of all ages and fitness levels, and can be easily modified to suit individual needs and preferences. So whether you're looking to improve your posture, reduce tension and stiffness in your upper body, or simply enjoy a greater sense of openness and ease in your chest and shoulders, these chair yoga exercises are a great place to start.

Here are a few chair yoga exercises to help open and stretch the chest:

EXERCISE 13: SEATED CHEST EXPANSION

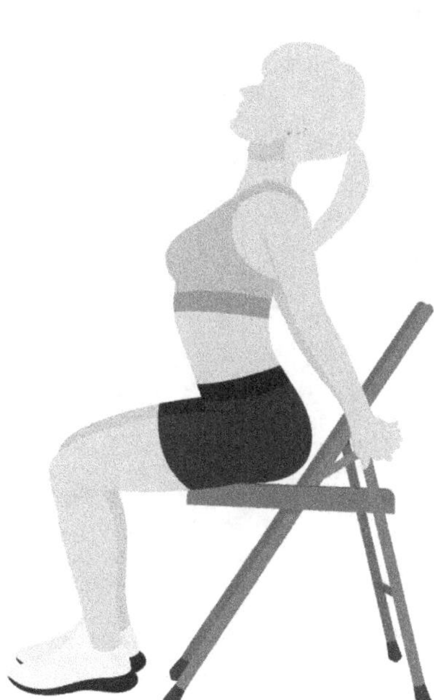

The seated chest expansion is a simple yet effective way to open and stretch the chest, shoulders, and upper back. By inhaling deeply and sweeping the arms back behind you, this exercise helps to counteract the effects of hunching and slouching, promoting better posture and alignment. Regularly practicing seated chest expansions can help to increase lung capacity and oxygenation while also relieving tension and stiffness in the shoulders and neck.

Here are some instructions to follow:

1. Sit up tall in your chair, with your feet flat on the floor and your arms extended out to the sides at shoulder height.
2. As you inhale, sweep your arms back behind you, squeezing your shoulder blades together and expanding your chest.
3. As you exhale, release your arms back to your sides.

4. Continue sweeping your arms back on your inhales and releasing them on your exhales for 5-10 breaths, moving slowly and smoothly with your breath.

Tips for Seated Chest Expansion:

- Keep your movements slow and gentle, avoiding any jerky or forceful motions.
- Focus on coordinating your movement with your breath, inhaling as you sweep your arms back and exhaling as you release them.
- If you have any shoulder pain or injuries, move cautiously and avoid any positions that cause discomfort.

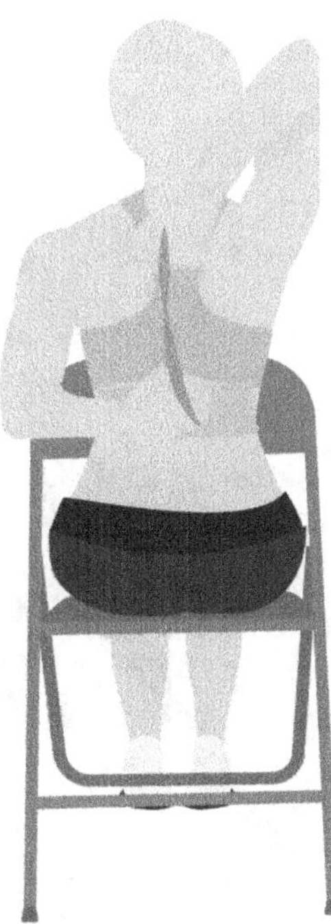

Seated cow face arms, also known as Gomukhasana arms, are a deep shoulder and upper back stretch that can help release tension and improve mobility in the shoulders. By reaching one arm overhead and the other behind your back, this exercise helps to open and stretch the chest, shoulders, and upper back, promoting better posture and alignment. Regularly practicing seated cow face arms can help to relieve tension and stiffness in the shoulders and neck while also improving overall upper body mobility and function.

Here are some instructions to follow:

1. Sit up tall in your chair, with your feet flat on the floor and your right arm extended overhead.
2. Bend your right elbow and reach your right hand down behind your back, between your shoulder blades.
3. Extend your left arm out to the side, then bend your left elbow and reach your left hand up behind your back, trying to clasp your hands together (if possible). If you can't clasp your hands together, you can use a strap or towel to bridge the gap between your hands.
4. Hold the pose for 3-5 breaths, focusing on breathing deeply and relaxing your shoulders away from your ears.
5. To release the pose, gently unclasp your hands (or release the strap/towel) and extend your arms back to your sides.
6. Repeat the pose on the other side, reaching your left arm overhead and your right arm behind your back, holding for 3-5 breaths before releasing.

Tips for Seated Cow Face Arms:

- Keep your shoulders relaxed and your elbows close to your head throughout the pose.
- If you have any shoulder pain or injuries, move cautiously and avoid any positions that cause discomfort.
- Use a strap or towel to bridge the gap between your hands if you can't clasp them together comfortably.

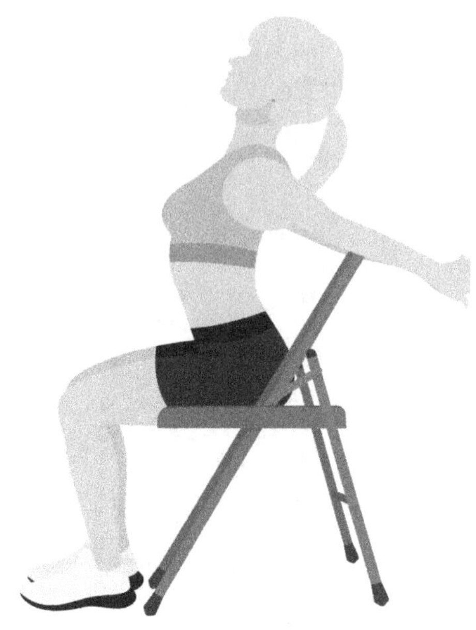

The seated chest opener is a simple yet effective way to open and stretch the chest and front of the shoulders. By interlacing your fingers behind your head and gently squeezing your shoulder blades together, this exercise helps to counteract the effects of rounding and hunching in the upper back, promoting better posture and alignment. Regularly practicing seated chest openers can help to increase lung capacity and promote deeper breathing while also improving overall upper body mobility and function.

1. Sit tall in your chair with your feet flat on the floor, hip-width apart.
2. Bring your hands behind your head, interlacing your fingers.
3. Gently squeeze your shoulder blades together and lift your chest upward.
4. Hold for 3-5 breaths, then release and bring your hands back to your lap.

Tips:
- Keep your core engaged and your spine straight throughout the pose.
- Avoid pulling on your head or neck; focus on lifting your chest and squeezing your shoulder blades.

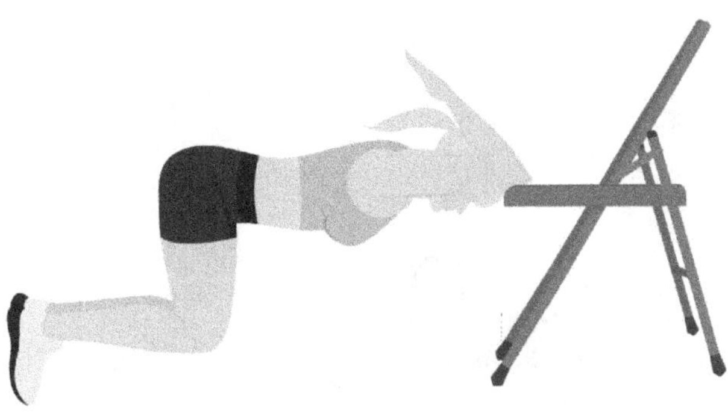

Seated puppy pose is a gentle yet effective way to stretch the chest, shoulders, and upper back. Walking your hands forward and hinging at your hips helps to open and stretch the entire upper body, promoting better posture and alignment. Regularly practicing seated puppy pose can help to relieve tension and stiffness in the upper body while also promoting a gentle inversion that can help to reduce stress and fatigue.

1. Stand in front of the chair and kneel with your feet flat on the floor, hip-width apart.
2. Place your hands on the seat of the chair, shoulder-width apart.
3. Walk with your hands forward, pivoting at your hips, raising your pelvis and lowering your chest towards your thighs.
4. Keep your arms straight and your shoulders relaxed, feeling the stretch in your chest and upper back.
5. Hold for 3-5 breaths, then walk your hands back and return to an upright seated position.

Tips:
- Keep your core engaged and your hips firmly planted in the chair throughout the pose.
- If you feel any strain in your lower back, bend your knees slightly or place a cushion on your thighs for support.

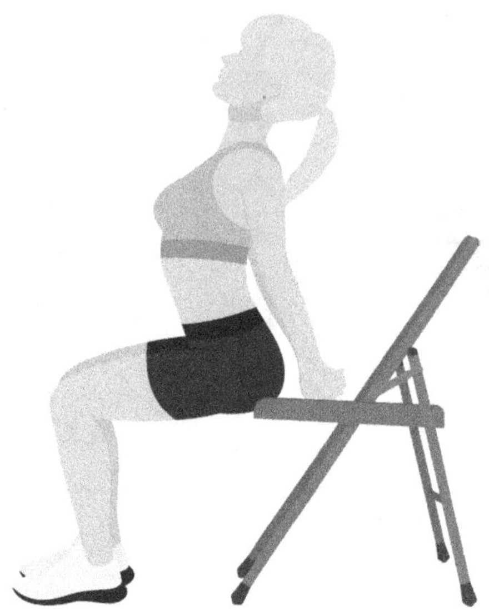

The seated supported fish pose is a gentle backbend that helps to open and stretch the chest, throat, and front of the shoulders. By pressing your hands into the seat of the chair and lifting your chest, this exercise helps to counteract the effects of slouching and promotes better posture and alignment. Regularly practicing seated supported fish poses can help stimulate the thyroid gland and promote healthy breathing while also improving overall upper body mobility and function.

1. Sit tall in your chair with your feet flat on the floor, hip-width apart.
2. Place your hands on the seat of the chair, fingers pointing toward your hips.
3. Press into your hands and lift your chest, tilting your head back slightly.
4. Hold for 3-5 breaths, then release and return to an upright seated position.

Tips:

- Keep your core engaged and your spine lifted throughout the pose.
- If you feel any strain in your neck or shoulders, reduce the amount of backbend or stop the exercise.

The legs are the foundation of our bodies, and keeping them strong and flexible is crucial for maintaining mobility, balance, and overall well-being as we age. However, many people tend to neglect their leg muscles, especially if they spend a lot of time sitting or have limited mobility. This can lead to stiffness, weakness, and even pain in the lower body, which can greatly impact one's quality of life.

Fortunately, chair yoga offers a variety of gentle yet effective exercises that can help to stretch and strengthen the legs, even for those with limited mobility or flexibility. By incorporating these exercises into your daily routine, you can improve your leg strength, flexibility, and circulation while also reducing stiffness and pain. These exercises are suitable for people of all ages and fitness levels and can be easily modified to suit individual needs and abilities.

Here are a few chair yoga exercises to help stretch and strengthen the legs:

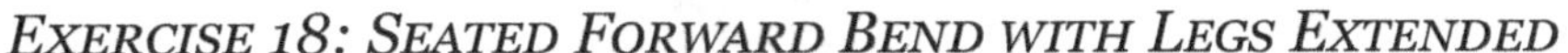

EXERCISE 18: SEATED FORWARD BEND WITH LEGS EXTENDED

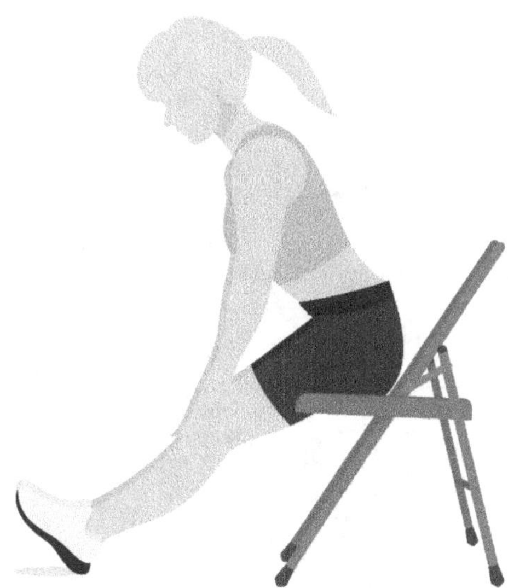

The seated forward bend with legs extended is a great way to stretch the hamstrings, calves, and lower back. By hinging forward at the hips and reaching for the toes, this exercise helps to lengthen the muscles in the back of the legs while also promoting good posture and spinal alignment. Regularly practicing seated forward bends can help to improve flexibility and mobility in the legs and hips while also calming the mind and reducing stress and anxiety.

Here's how to do it:

1. Sit up tall in your chair, with your legs extended out in front of you and your feet flexed.
2. As you inhale, lengthen your spine and lift your chest.
3. As you exhale, hinge forward at your hips, reaching your hands towards your toes. Keep your back straight and your core engaged, and only go as far as feels comfortable for you.
4. Hold the stretch for 3-5 breaths, focusing on breathing deeply and relaxing into the stretch.
5. To release the stretch, inhale and slowly roll up to a seated position, stacking your vertebrae one at a time.

Tips for Seated Forward Bend with Legs Extended:
- Keep your back straight and your core engaged throughout the stretch, avoiding any rounding in your spine.
- Only go as far as feels comfortable for you, and never force or strain to reach your toes.
- If you have any lower back pain or injuries, move cautiously and avoid any positions that cause discomfort.

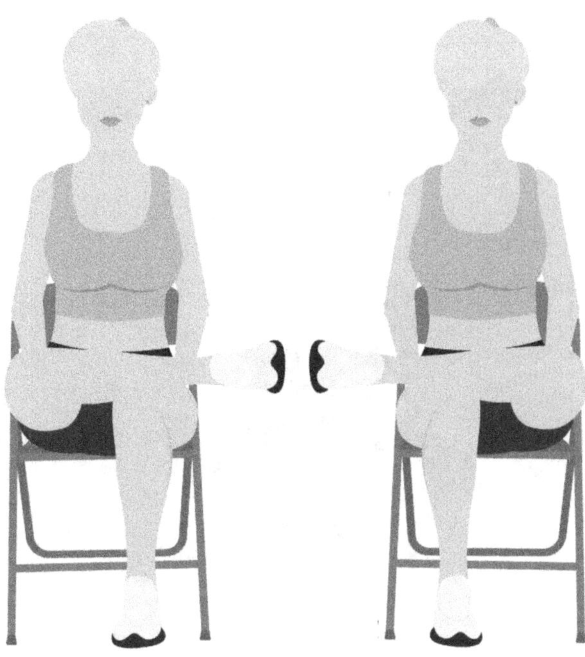

The seated pigeon pose is a deep hip opener that can help to release tension and improve mobility in the hips and lower back. Crossing one ankle over the opposite thigh and gently pressing the knee down helps to stretch the glutes and outer hips while also promoting good posture and alignment. Regularly practicing seated pigeon poses can help to relieve tension and stiffness in the lower body while also improving overall hip mobility and range of motion.

Here's how to do it:

1. Sit up tall in your chair with your feet flat on the floor.
2. Cross your right ankle over your left thigh, just above your knee.
3. Gently press down on your right knee with your right hand, feeling the stretch in your right hip and glutes.
4. Hold the stretch for 3-5 breaths, focusing on breathing deeply and relaxing into the stretch.
5. To release the stretch, gently uncross your right leg and return your foot to the floor.
6. Repeat the stretch on the other side, crossing your left ankle over your right thigh and holding for 3-5 breaths before releasing.

Tips for Seated Pigeon Pose:

- Keep your back straight and your core engaged throughout the stretch, avoiding any rounding in your spine.
- Only go as far as feels comfortable for you, and never force or strain to deepen the stretch.
- If you have any hip pain or injuries, move cautiously and avoid any positions that cause discomfort.

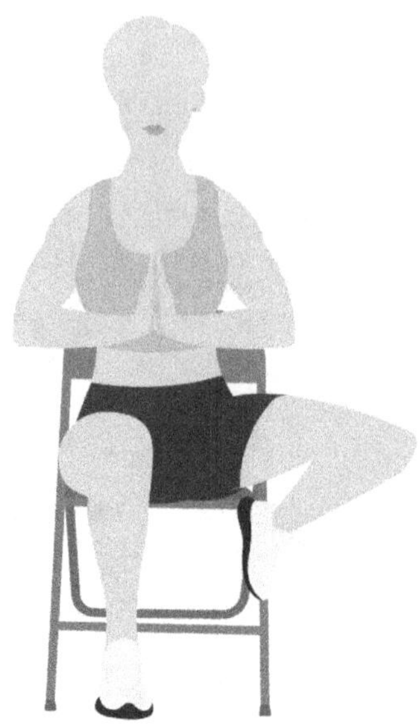

The seated tree pose is a great way to improve balance, stability, and focus while also strengthening the legs and core. By placing one foot against the opposite inner thigh and pressing the foot and thigh together, this exercise helps to create resistance and stability while also promoting good posture and alignment. Regularly practicing seated tree pose can help to improve overall balance and coordination while also reducing stress and anxiety.

Here's how to do it:

1. Sit up tall in your chair with your feet flat on the floor.
2. Lift your right foot and place the sole of your foot against your left inner thigh (or wherever is comfortable for you).
3. Press your foot gently into your thigh and your thigh back into your foot to create resistance and stability.
4. Bring your hands to prayer position in front of your chest, or rest them on your thighs.
5. Hold the pose for 3-5 breaths, focusing on breathing deeply and maintaining your balance.
6. To release the pose, gently lower your right foot back to the floor.
7. Repeat the pose on the other side, lifting your left foot and holding for 3-5 breaths before releasing.

Tips for Seated Tree Pose:

- Keep your back straight and your core engaged throughout the pose, avoiding any slouching or rounding in your spine.
- To assist you in staying balanced, concentrate your eyes on a stationary spot in front of you.
- If you have any knee pain or injuries, move cautiously and avoid any positions that cause discomfort.

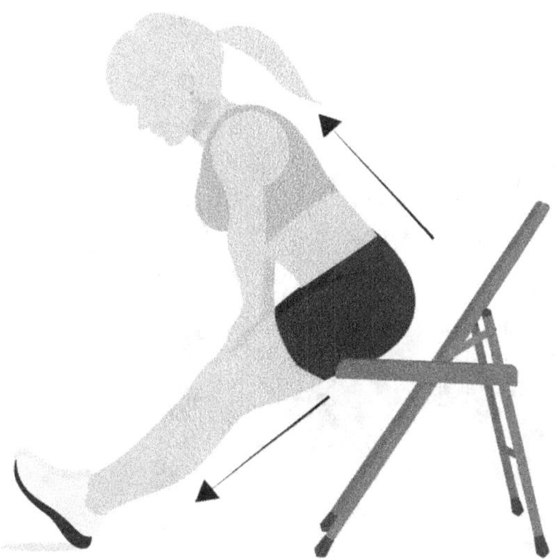

The seated hamstring stretch is a simple yet effective way to stretch the back of the legs and improve flexibility in the lower body. By extending one leg forward and hinging at the hips to reach for the toes, this exercise helps to lengthen the hamstrings and calves while also relieving tension and stiffness in the lower back and legs.

1. Sit tall in your chair with your right foot flat on the floor and your left leg extended, heel resting on the floor.
2. Hinge forward at your hips, keeping your back straight and reaching for your left toes.
3. Hold for 3-5 breaths, then release and repeat on the opposite side.

Tips:

- Keep your core engaged and your spine straight throughout the stretch.
- If you can't reach your toes, place your hands on your thighs or use a strap around your foot.

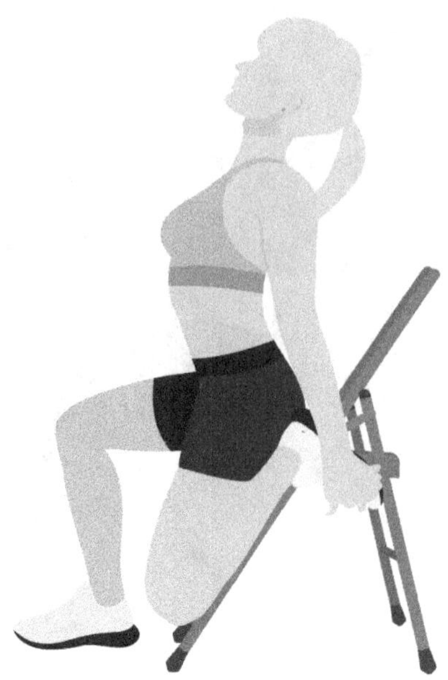

Seated Hero's Pose offers numerous benefits for seniors practicing chair yoga. By targeting the quadriceps and hip flexors, this posture helps to alleviate tightness and stiffness in these areas, promoting better mobility and flexibility. Additionally, Virasana can help improve circulation in the legs, reduce the risk of developing blood clots, and alleviate discomfort associated with prolonged sitting. As with all chair yoga postures, it is essential to listen to your body and only stretch within your comfortable range of motion, modifying the pose as needed to suit your individual needs and abilities.

INSTRUCTIONS:

1. Begin by shifting to the side of your chair, allowing your right leg to hang off the chair.
2. Hold the edge of your chair firmly with your left hand for support and stability.
3. Lean slightly to the left as you bend your right knee, bringing your right heel towards your buttock.
4. Reach down with your right hand and take hold of your right foot. If this proves challenging, you can use a strap or a towel to loop around your foot, making it easier to grasp.
5. Gently pull your heel closer to your buttock, focusing on feeling a stretch in the front of your right thigh. If you experience any discomfort or sensations in your knee, release your foot slightly until you find a comfortable stretch.
6. Hold the pose for 3-5 breaths, allowing your muscles to relax and lengthen with each exhalation.
7. To release the pose, slowly let go of your foot and allow your right leg to return to its original position.
8. Repeat the process on the left side, shifting to the side of your chair and bending your left knee to take hold of your left foot.

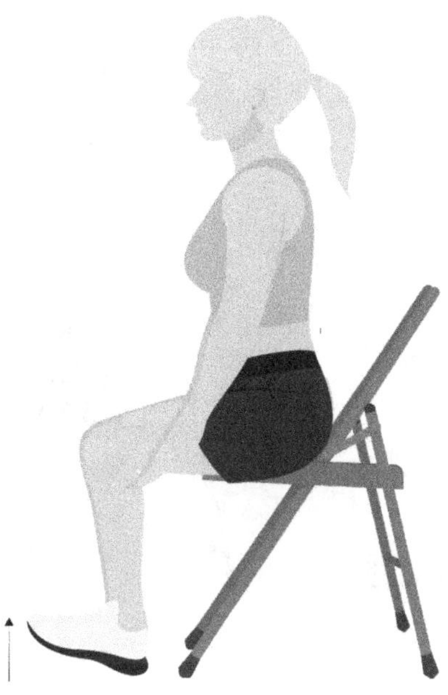

Seated foot and ankle rolls are a simple way to improve mobility and flexibility in the feet and ankles while also increasing blood circulation in the lower legs. By making circular motions with the feet and ankles, this exercise helps to relieve tension and stiffness while also promoting overall foot and ankle health.

1. Sit tall in your chair with your feet flat on the floor, hip-width apart.
2. Lift your right foot off the floor and begin making circular motions with your ankle.
3. Perform 10 circles in each direction, then repeat on the left foot.

Tips:

- Keep your core engaged and your spine straight throughout the exercise.
- If you experience any pain or discomfort, reduce the size of the circles or stop the exercise.

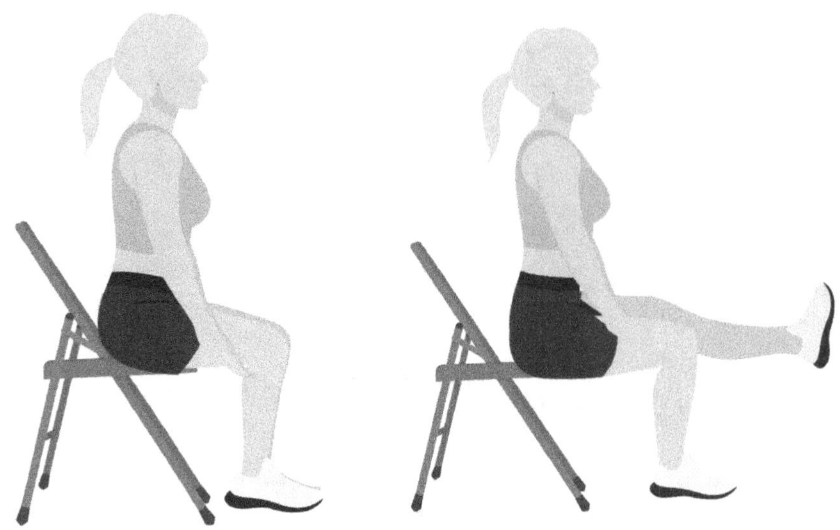

Seated leg lifts are a great way to strengthen the quadriceps and hip flexors while also improving stability and balance in the lower body. By lifting one leg at a time and holding it in an extended position, this exercise helps to engage the muscles in the front of the thighs while also increasing blood circulation in the legs.

1. Sit tall in your chair with your feet flat on the floor, hip-width apart.
2. Lift your right leg, extending it forward and keeping your foot flexed.
3. Hold for 3-5 breaths, then lower your leg back to the floor and repeat on the left side.

Tips:

- Keep your core engaged and your spine straight throughout the exercise.
- If you feel any strain in your lower back, reduce the height of your leg lift or stop the exercise.

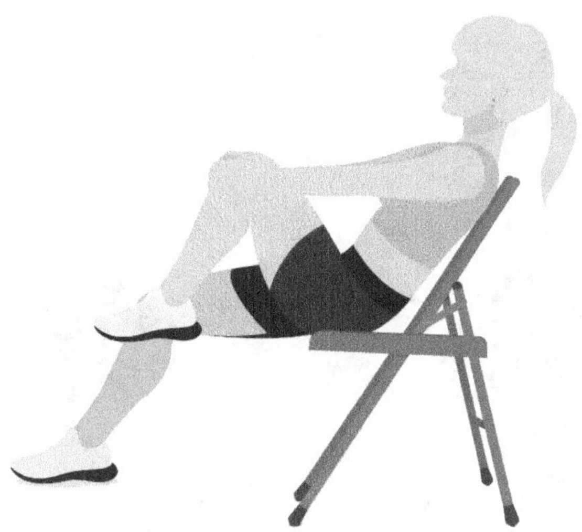

The seated knee-to-chest stretch is a gentle way to release tension and improve mobility in the hips, glutes, and lower back. Hugging one knee at a time towards the chest helps to stretch the muscles in the hips and buttocks while also promoting good posture and spinal alignment.

1. Sit tall in your chair with your feet flat on the floor, hip-width apart.
2. Lift your right knee toward your chest, grasping your shin with both hands.
3. Gently pull your knee closer to your chest, feeling the stretch in your hip and lower back.
4. Hold for 3-5 breaths, then release and repeat on the left side.

Tips:
- Keep your core engaged and your spine straight throughout the pose.
- If you feel any pain or discomfort, reduce the pressure on your knee or stop the exercise.

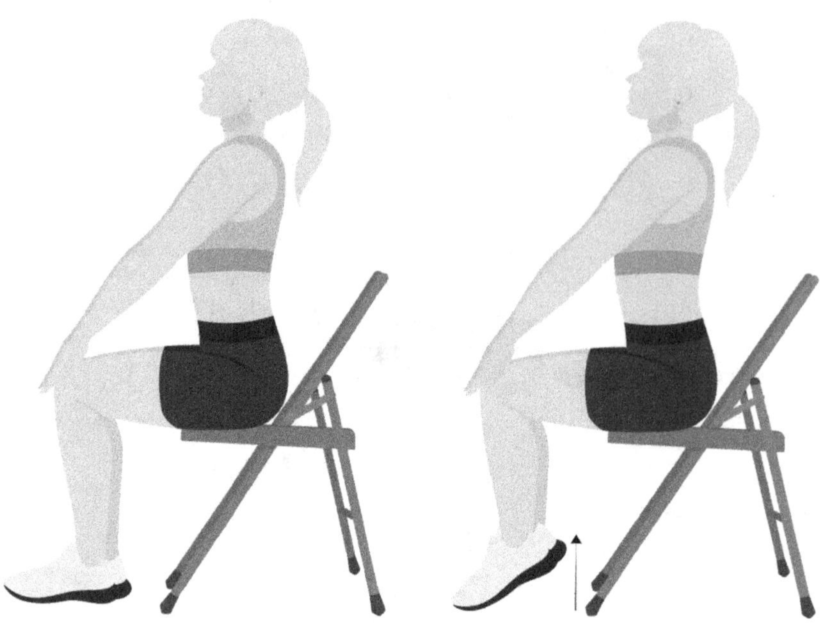

Seated calf raises are a simple way to strengthen the calves and ankles while also improving stability and balance in the lower legs. By lifting the heels off the ground and holding them for a few breaths, this exercise helps to engage the muscles in the back of the lower legs while also increasing blood circulation in the feet and ankles.

1. Sit tall in your chair with your feet flat on the floor, hip-width apart.
2. Lift your heels off the floor, coming onto the balls of your feet.
3. Hold for 3-5 breaths, then lower your heels back to the floor.
4. Repeat for 10-15 repetitions.

Tips:

- Keep your core engaged and your spine straight throughout the exercise.
- If you feel any strain or discomfort in your feet or ankles, reduce the range of motion or stop the exercise.

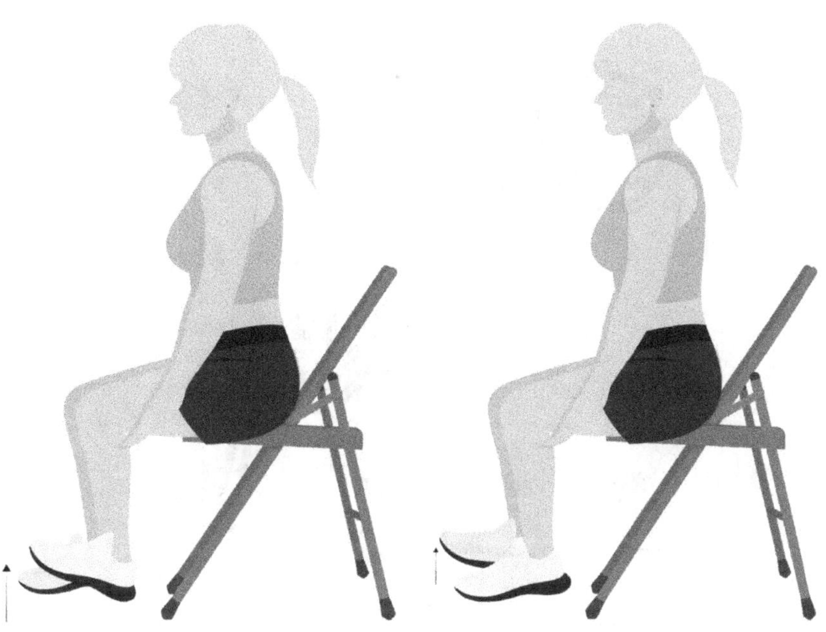

Seated toe taps are a gentle way to improve coordination and agility in the feet and legs while also providing a mild cardiovascular workout. Alternately tapping the toes on the ground helps to engage the muscles in the feet and lower legs while also increasing blood flow and circulation.

1. Sit tall in your chair with your feet flat on the floor, hip-width apart.
2. Lift your right foot off the floor and tap your toes on the ground.
3. Alternate tapping your right and left toes on the floor as if you were marching in place.
4. Continue for 30-60 seconds.

Tips:

- Keep your core engaged and your spine straight throughout the exercise.
- If you feel any pain or discomfort, reduce the speed or height of your toe taps or stop the exercise.

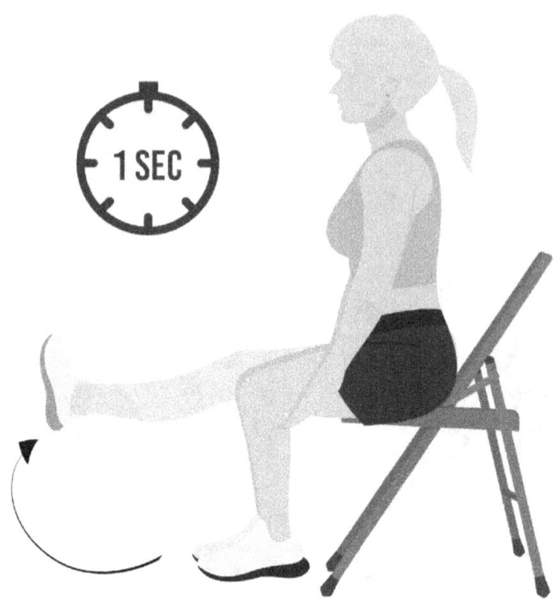

Seated leg extensions are a great way to strengthen the quadriceps and hip flexors while also improving stability and control in the lower body. By extending one leg at a time and holding it in a straight position, this exercise helps to engage the muscles in the front of the thighs while also promoting good posture and alignment.

1. Sit tall in your chair with your feet flat on the floor, hip-width apart.
2. Lift your right leg, extending it forward and keeping your foot flexed.
3. Slowly lower your leg back to the floor, then repeat on the left side.
4. Alternate legs for 10-15 repetitions on each side.

Tips:
- Keep your core engaged and your spine straight throughout the exercise.
- If you feel any strain in your lower back or knees, reduce the height of your leg lift or stop the exercise.

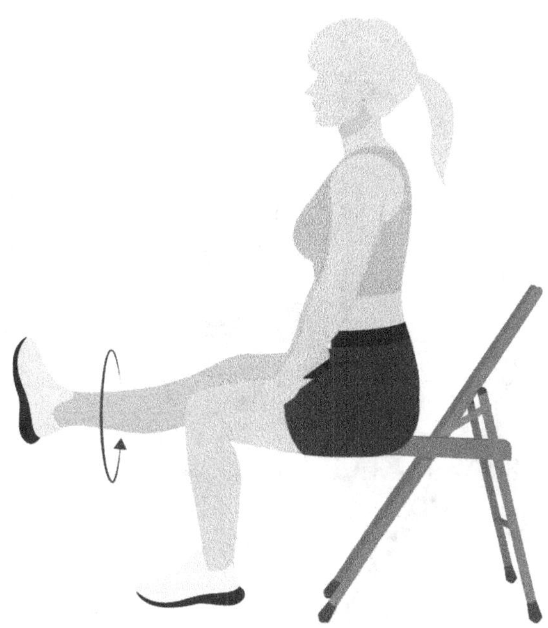

Seated leg circles are a simple way to improve mobility and flexibility in the hips and legs while also increasing blood circulation in the lower body. By making circular motions with one leg at a time, this exercise helps to stretch and strengthen the muscles in the hips and thighs while also promoting overall leg health.

1. Sit tall in your chair with your feet flat on the floor, hip-width apart.
2. Lift your right leg, extending it forward and keeping your foot flexed.
3. Begin making small circular motions with your leg, gradually increasing the size of the circles.
4. Perform 10 circles in each direction, then repeat on the left leg.

Tips:

- Keep your core engaged and your spine straight throughout the exercise.
- If you experience any pain or discomfort, reduce the size of the circles or stop the exercise.

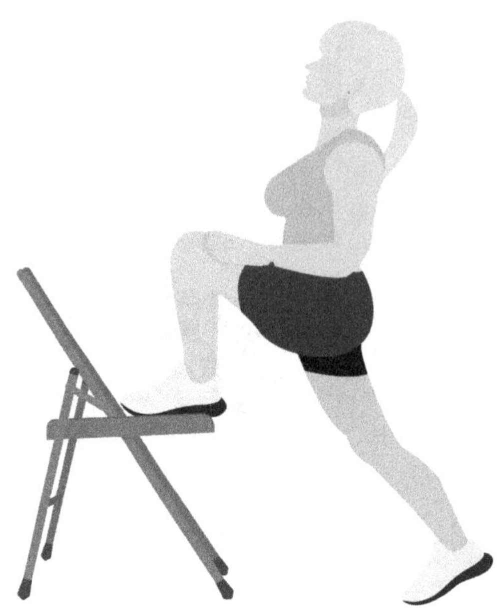

The Chair Yoga Lunge Pose offers several benefits for seniors. By stretching the calves and hip flexors, this posture can help improve flexibility and range of motion in the lower body. Additionally, the lunge position helps to strengthen the legs, particularly the quadriceps and glutes, which are essential for maintaining balance and stability. Practicing this pose regularly can also help alleviate stiffness and discomfort in the legs and hips, promoting better overall mobility and function. As with all chair yoga postures, it is crucial to listen to your body and only move within a comfortable range, using the chair for support and stability as needed.

INSTRUCTIONS:

1. Begin by standing in front of your chair, approximately an arm's length away, facing the seat of the chair.
2. If you have concerns about balance, turn the chair 90 degrees so that you can hold onto the back of the chair for added support.
3. Shift your weight onto your left foot, ensuring that it is firmly planted on the ground.
4. Carefully step up onto the chair with your right foot, placing it flat on the seat of the chair.
5. Lean forward towards your front leg (the right leg on the chair), keeping your torso upright and your core engaged. You may feel a stretch in the back of your left calf and the front of your right hip.
6. Pay close attention to your right knee, ensuring that it remains directly above your right ankle and does not extend forward beyond your toes.
7. Hold this position for 3-5 breaths, focusing on maintaining balance and feeling the stretch in your legs and hips.
8. To release the pose, slowly step your right foot back down to the ground, returning to a standing position.
9. Repeat the process on the other side, stepping up with your left foot and keeping your right foot on the ground.

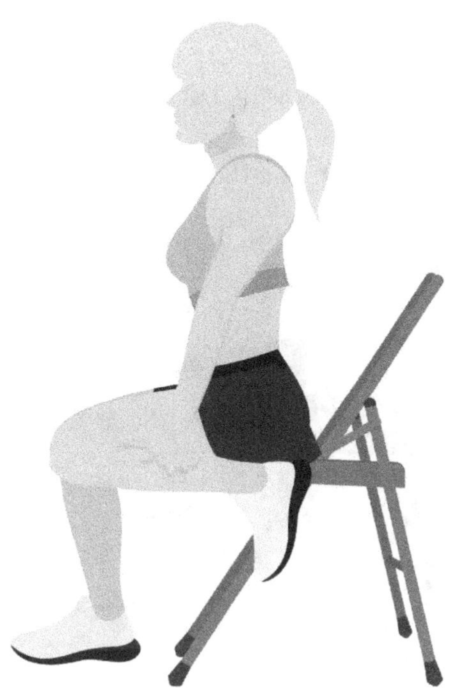

The Half Supine Pose offers numerous benefits for seniors practicing chair yoga. By targeting the thighs and hips, this posture helps to alleviate tension and stiffness in these areas, promoting better flexibility and range of motion. Regular practice of Ardha Supta Virasana can also help improve circulation in the legs, reduce the risk of developing cramps or blood clots, and ease discomfort associated with prolonged sitting. Additionally, this pose can help promote a sense of relaxation and stress relief, as it encourages deep breathing and a focus on releasing tension in the lower body. As with all chair yoga postures, it is essential to listen to your body and only move within a comfortable range, modifying the pose as needed to suit your individual needs and abilities.

INSTRUCTIONS:

1. Begin by sitting upright in your chair, with your feet flat on the ground and your hands holding the sides of the chair for support.
2. Take a deep breath in, and as you exhale, bend your right leg, bringing your right heel towards the back of the chair. If needed, you can use your right hand to help lift and guide your leg into position.
3. If possible, bring your right heel to rest on the chair seat beside your right hip. If this is challenging, simply continue to hold your right foot with your right hand, keeping your leg bent.
4. Throughout the pose, maintain a straight spine, keeping your head, neck, and trunk in alignment. Avoid slouching or rounding your back.
5. Hold the position for 3-5 breaths, focusing on relaxing your right thigh and hip muscles with each exhalation.
6. To release the pose, gently lower your right leg back to the ground, allowing it to rest alongside your left leg.
7. Repeat the process on the left side, bending your left leg and bringing your left heel towards the back of the chair.

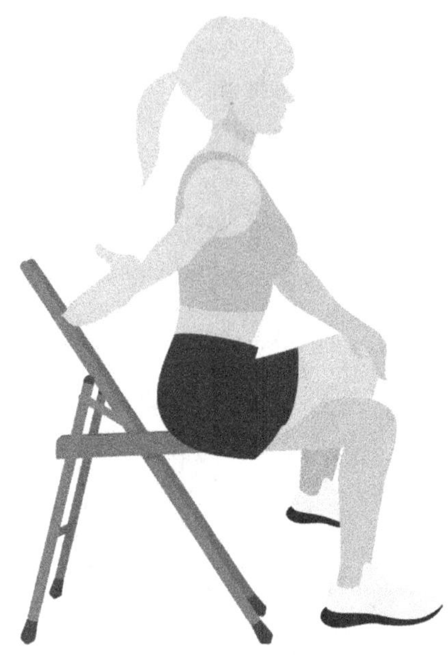

Seated eagle legs are a challenging balance pose that helps to stretch the hips, glutes, and outer thighs while also improving focus and concentration. By crossing one thigh over the other and wrapping the foot behind the calf (if possible), this exercise creates a deep stretch in the hips and buttocks while also promoting good posture and alignment.

1. Sit tall in your chair with your feet flat on the floor, hip-width apart.
2. Cross your right thigh over your left thigh, and if possible, wrap your right foot behind your left calf.
3. Gently press your thighs together, feeling the stretch in your hips and outer thighs.
4. Hold for 3-5 breaths, then release and repeat on the opposite side.

Tips:
- Keep your core engaged and your spine straight throughout the pose.
- If you can't wrap your foot behind your calf, simply cross your thighs and rest your top foot on your bottom thigh.

Chapter 9

Improving Mobility Positions: Tips and Techniques for Seniors

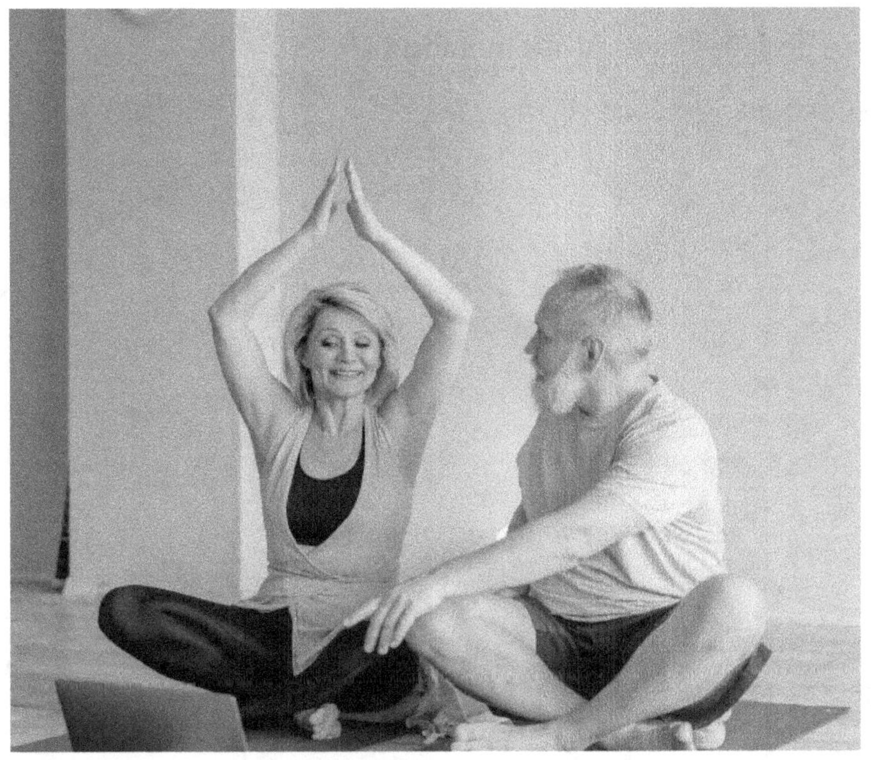

Mobility is the key to staying active and independent as we age. Whether it's reaching for a high shelf, bending down to tie our shoes, or simply getting up from a chair, having good mobility makes daily life easier and more enjoyable. Mobility positions, such as those found in yoga and other gentle exercises, play a crucial role in maintaining and enhancing mobility as we grow older. In this guide, we'll explore practical tips and techniques to help seniors improve their mobility positions, enabling them to move with greater ease and comfort.

In simpler words, Mobility positions in yoga for seniors are all about moving your body in ways that help you stay flexible, strong, and balanced. As we get older, our bodies might not move as easily as they used to. That's where mobility positions come in—they're like little stretches and movements that help keep your body feeling good and working well. In this guide, we'll take a closer look at what mobility positions are, why they're important for seniors, and some simple examples you can try at home.

What Are Mobility Positions?

Think of mobility positions as gentle movements and stretches designed to keep your body limber and agile. They're not about doing crazy yoga poses or bending yourself into a pretzel. Instead, they focus on helping you move better in your everyday life. These positions can target different parts of your body, like your neck, shoulders, back, hips, and legs, helping to improve flexibility, strength, and balance.

Why Are Mobility Positions Important for Seniors?

With age, our bodies tend to become less flexible and strong, which can complicate everyday activities such as bending down to lace up sneakers or stretching to retrieve items from elevated places. Engaging in mobility exercises can mitigate these effects by softly stretching and fortifying the muscles and joints. They also help improve circulation and reduce stiffness, which can make it easier to move around and stay active as you age. Additionally, regular practice of mobility exercises can enhance balance and coordination, which helps in reducing the risk of falls and injuries.

As we age, it's common to experience a decrease in mobility and flexibility, which can make everyday tasks more challenging and increase the risk of falls and injuries. Practicing chair yoga regularly can help improve mobility and flexibility, making it easier to move through life with ease and confidence.

Here are four chair yoga exercises designed to improve mobility:

EXERCISE 33: SIDE ANGLE POSE

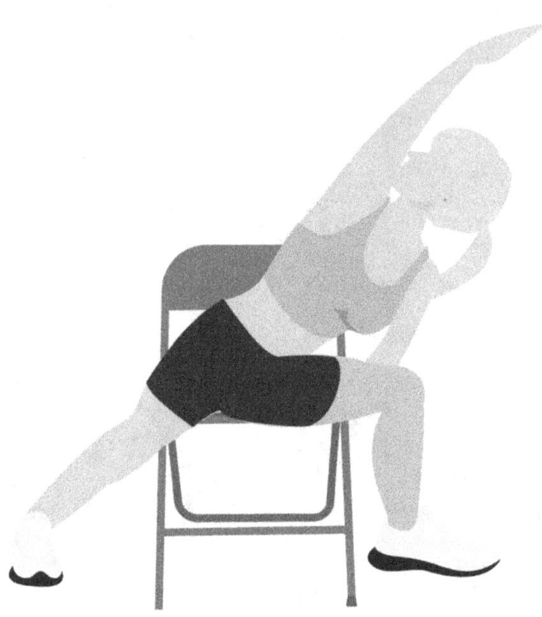

The Side Angle Pose, or Utthita Parsvakonasana, is a powerful and dynamic chair yoga posture that offers a multitude of benefits for both the body and mind. This pose deeply stretches and strengthens the legs, hips, and ankles while also opening the chest and shoulders, promoting better posture and breathing. As you side bend your torso and extend your arm overhead, you'll experience a lovely lengthening of the spine and a gentle twist, which can help to improve spinal mobility and flexibility. Holding this pose also requires balance and stability, helping to enhance your overall sense of grounding and focus. Consistently performing the Side Angle Pose can boost energy levels, alleviate stress and tension, and enhance overall well-being.

1. Sit upright in a chair, ensuring your feet are flat on the floor and spaced hip-width apart.
2. Stretch your right leg to the side while keeping your foot grounded.
3. Bend your right knee so it aligns with your right ankle, ensuring your right thigh is parallel to the ground.
4. Raise your left arm towards the ceiling, then lean your upper body to the right.
5. Position your right elbow on your right thigh, or for more stretch, place your right hand on the floor outside your right foot.
6. Reach your left arm over your head, aiming to form a straight line from your left foot to your left fingertips.
7. Turn your gaze upwards towards your left hand, or keep it forward if that feels better.
8. Maintain this pose for 3-5 breaths, concentrating on stretching your spine and expanding your chest.

9. To exit the pose, inhale and return your torso to the center. Lower your left arm and straighten your right leg.
10. Switch to the other side and repeat the process.

Tips:

- Engage your core to maintain stability and prevent sagging into your right side.
- If you experience tightness in your hips, use a folded blanket or a block beneath your right sitting bone for additional support.

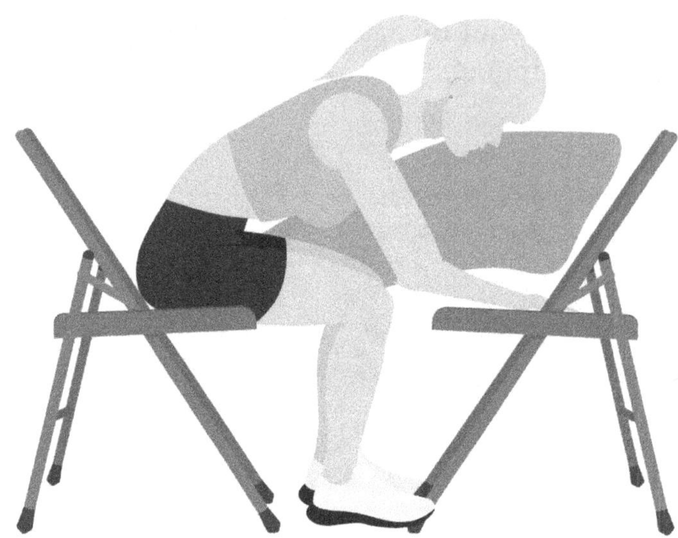

The Child's Pose offers numerous benefits, including the relief of back pain, improved spinal flexibility, and reduced stress and anxiety. This pose is particularly advantageous for seniors, as it can be easily incorporated into a daily routine, even performed on a bed just after waking up. By sitting upright with legs tucked under the buttocks and gently bending forward onto the bed, one can experience an instant sense of refreshment and rejuvenation. As with all yoga postures, it is essential to listen to your body, move within your comfortable range, and use props as needed to ensure a safe and beneficial practice.

INSTRUCTIONS:

1. Begin by sitting deep into your chair, with your feet hip-width apart and your hands resting on your knees. Ensure that your spine is straight, and sit tall as if gently pushing the crown of your head towards the ceiling.

2. Be mindful not to slouch, and slowly start bending forward. Pay close attention to the sensations in your body as you progress. If you feel any resistance in your spine, hips, or neck, pause, take a deep breath, and assess whether to continue or return to an upright position. If needed, perform a few warm-up exercises before attempting the pose again.

3. Allow your hands to stretch straight ahead as you bend forward, aiming to rest your chest on your thighs. Keep your spine elongated, imagining that you are pushing an invisible object forward with the crown of your head. This visualization helps ensure that you achieve the maximum comfortable extension in your spine. You may choose to lower your hands and let them hang by your sides, touch the ground, or cross them under your thighs for added support and to hold the position longer.

4. If you have chronic back pain or require additional support, consider placing blocks under your legs to raise your knees. Position the blocks before beginning the pose to ensure a comfortable and stable foundation. This modification can help you achieve the desired forward bend more easily.

5. For those who need extra support or wish to maintain the pose for an extended period,

place another chair facing you, about a foot in front. This chair can serve as a surface for your hands to rest upon, allowing you to sustain the pose comfortably.

6. Remember that the Child's Pose is meant to be extremely relaxing and provide instant relief to stiff bones and muscles. Once you have held the pose for your desired duration, slowly release and return to an upright seated position.

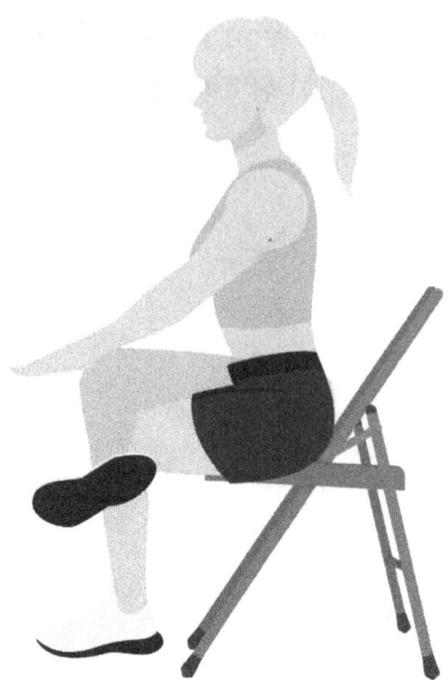

The seated figure-4 stretch is a deep hip opener that can help improve mobility and flexibility in the hips and lower back. By crossing one ankle over the opposite thigh and gently pressing down on the knee, this stretch targets the muscles and connective tissue in the hips and glutes, helping to release tension and tightness. The seated figure-4 stretch is effective in enhancing posture and alignment by promoting a neutral pelvic position and elongating the spine. This is especially beneficial for individuals who spend extended periods seated, as it helps counter the impacts of sustained hip flexion.

Here's how to perform the stretch:

1. Sit erect in your chair, ensuring your feet are flat on the ground.
2. Place your right ankle on your left thigh, forming a "figure-4" with your legs.
3. Use your right hand to lightly press your right knee downward, experiencing a stretch in your right hip and buttocks.
4. To intensify the stretch, lean forward from your hips, maintaining a straight back and an engaged core.
5. Maintain the position for 3-5 breaths, concentrating on deep breathing and easing into the stretch.
6. To end the stretch, carefully lower your right leg and place your foot back on the floor.
7. Perform the stretch on the opposite side by crossing your left ankle over your right thigh, holding for 3-5 breaths before gently releasing.

Tips for Seated Figure-4 Stretch:

- Maintain a straight back and keep your core active during the stretch, ensuring there is no rounding of your spine.
- Progress in the stretch only to the extent that is comfortable for you, and avoid pushing or straining to deepen it further.
- If you have any hip pain or injuries, move cautiously and avoid any positions that cause discomfort.

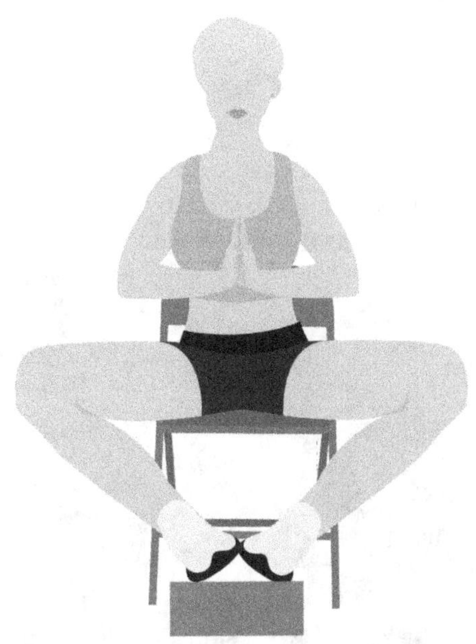

The Seated Butterfly Pose offers numerous benefits for seniors practicing chair yoga. By targeting the muscles of the pelvis and inner thighs, this posture helps to strengthen the pelvic floor, which can improve bladder control, reduce the risk of incontinence, and alleviate lower back pain. Additionally, the gentle flapping motion of the legs helps to improve circulation, reduce stiffness, and promote overall flexibility in the hips and thighs.

Instructions:

1. Start in Mountain Pose by sitting with your feet firmly planted on the ground and your hands resting on your knees. Keep your spine aligned, and your shoulders relaxed.
2. With your right hand, carefully raise your right foot and set it on the chair seat, positioning the sole of your foot against the inner thigh of your left leg. Stabilize your body in this posture, keeping your back straight, and your shoulders spread wide.
3. Keeping your right hand grasping your right foot, begin to gently flap your right leg up and down as if imitating the movement of a butterfly's wings. Perform ten soft flaps, then slowly drop your right leg to the ground. Repeat the technique with the other leg.
4. Once you feel confident and comfortable with the single-leg butterfly, try lifting both legs simultaneously onto the chair seat. Grasp the soles of your feet together using your hands and softly flutter your legs up and down at the same time. Remember to keep your spine erect throughout the movement, avoiding any slouching or rounding of the back.
5. After completing about ten flaps with both legs, gently release your feet and allow your legs to return to the starting position. Take a moment to relax and observe any sensations in your body.

MUSCLE STRETCHING IMPROVEMENT POSITIONS

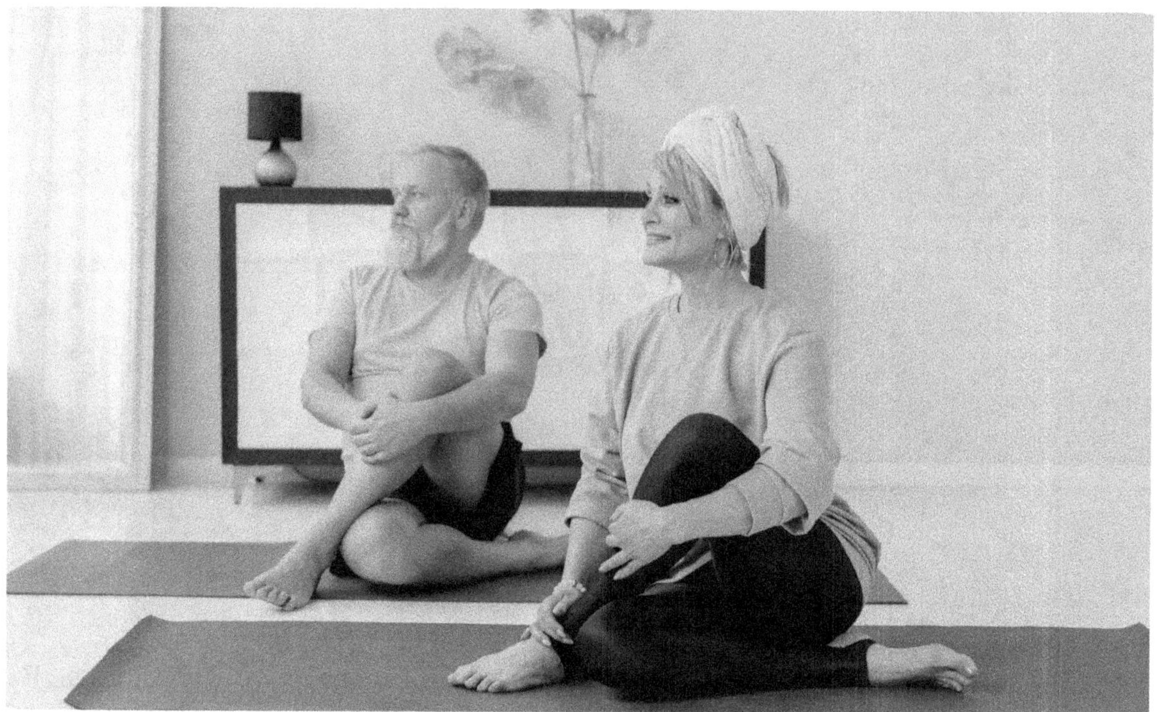

"Stretching is the key to unlock the body's potential for flexibility and strength."
- Arnold Schwarzenegger

Muscle stretching, often overlooked amidst the buzz of high-intensity workouts and flashy fitness trends, quietly holds the key to unlocking a world of physical freedom and vitality. It's not just a mundane task to check off your fitness checklist; rather, it's a profound practice that speaks to the very essence of human movement and well-being. In the realm of fitness and wellness, muscle stretching stands tall as a foundational pillar, offering a gateway to enhanced flexibility, improved range of motion, and a host of other benefits that transcend age, fitness level, and lifestyle.

Imagine your muscles as resilient yet pliable, strands of elastic waiting to be gently coaxed into expansion and lengthening. That's precisely the essence of muscle stretching—a simple yet potent practice that invites you to explore the full potential of your body's mobility. It's not about contorting yourself into impossible shapes or pushing your body beyond its limits; rather, it's about honoring your body's natural range of motion and gently encouraging it to reach new heights of flexibility and freedom.

Understanding Muscle Stretching:

Muscle stretching is the act of deliberately extending the muscles beyond their resting length, either statically or dynamically. This goal can be reached using several methods, such as static stretching, dynamic stretching, and proprioceptive neuromuscular facilitation (PNF). Regardless of the method used, the primary goal of muscle stretching is to improve flexibility and mobility by lengthening the muscles and increasing the range of motion around the joints.

Moreover, muscle stretching serves as a potent tool for injury prevention—a shield against the proverbial bumps and bruises that life may throw your way. Tight muscles are akin to dormant volcanoes, poised to erupt with the smallest trigger. However, through consistent stretching, you can neutralize these pockets of tension, lowering the likelihood of strains, sprains, and various musculoskeletal injuries.

Now, let's talk about performance—the holy grail of fitness enthusiasts and athletes alike. Whether you're a weekend warrior hitting the trails or a seasoned athlete aiming for gold, stretching can give you the edge you need to excel. Improved flexibility and range of motion mean more efficient movement patterns, smoother performance, and reduced risk of overuse injuries—qualities that can take your performance from mediocre to magnificent.

But perhaps the most underrated benefit of muscle stretching lies in its ability to soothe the soul and calm the mind. In a world that often feels like a whirlwind of chaos and stress, stretching offers a tranquil oasis—a moment of respite amidst the hustle and bustle of daily life. The slow, deliberate movements of stretching invite you to breathe deeply, center your thoughts, and reconnect with your body in a profound and meaningful way.

So, how can you harness the transformative power of muscle stretching in your daily life? It's simpler than you might think. Begin by setting aside a few minutes each day for stretching—whether it's early in the morning, during your lunch break, or just before you go to sleep. Focus on areas of tightness and tension, gently coaxing your muscles into relaxation and release. And remember, it's not about pushing yourself to the brink of discomfort; rather, it's about honoring your body's unique needs and limitations and embracing the journey of self-discovery and self-care.

In the grand tapestry of fitness and wellness, muscle stretching is the humble thread that binds it all together—a simple yet powerful practice that holds the key to unlocking your body's full potential. So, take a deep breath, reach for the sky, and let the transformative magic of stretching carry you to new heights of flexibility, freedom, and well-being.

Importance of Muscle Stretching

Why does muscle stretching matter, you might wonder? Well, let's peel back the layers and uncover the myriad reasons why this humble practice deserves a prime spot in your daily routine. Firstly, stretching acts as a lubricant for your muscles, akin to oiling the gears of a well-oiled machine. By elongating and lengthening the muscles, stretching helps to improve circulation, reduce muscle tension, and alleviate stiffness—a trifecta of benefits that can spell relief for anyone grappling with the aches and pains of daily life.

But the benefits of muscle stretching extend far beyond mere physical relief. Picture yourself standing tall and confident, moving through life with a sense of grace and ease. That's the power of improved flexibility and range of motion unlocked through regular stretching. Whether you're reaching for a jar on the top shelf, bending down to tie your shoelaces, or simply navigating the twists and turns of everyday life, flexible muscles, and joints are your silent companions, supporting you every step of the way.

Muscle stretching plays a crucial role in maintaining and enhancing overall physical health and well-being. Here are some key reasons why muscle stretching is important:

1. **Improves Flexibility:**

    One of the primary advantages of stretching muscles is the improvement in flexibility. Flexibility is the ability of a joint or series of joints to move freely, and maintaining good flexibility is crucial for carrying out daily activities effortlessly and minimizing injury risks. Regular muscle stretching enhances this flexibility and supports optimal joint functionality.

1. **Prevents Injury:**

   Tight muscles can restrict your body's movement range and lead to uneven muscle strength, which may increase injury risks. Stretching helps mitigate these issues by elongating the stiff muscles and easing tension, thus decreasing the chances of experiencing strains, sprains, and other types of soft tissue injuries.

1. **Relieves Muscle Tension and Soreness:**

   Factors such as exercise, poor posture, and stress can lead to muscle tension and soreness. Stretching plays a significant role in relieving this discomfort by enhancing blood circulation to the muscles. This not only helps in delivering essential nutrients and oxygen but also aids in the expulsion of metabolic wastes. The result is relaxed muscles, reduced soreness, and better overall mobility and comfort.

1. **Improves Posture:**

   Poor posture is a common problem that can lead to musculoskeletal issues such as back pain, neck pain, and headaches. Stretching muscles can assist in correcting postural imbalances by elongating muscles that are tight and strengthening those that are weak. By improving posture, stretching can alleviate discomfort and prevent long-term structural problems associated with poor alignment.

1. **Supports Joint Health:**

   Adequate joint mobility is essential for maintaining optimal function and preventing degenerative conditions such as osteoarthritis. Muscle stretching helps preserve joint health by improving flexibility and reducing stiffness, which can help prevent joint pain and dysfunction. Additionally, stretching promotes synovial fluid production, which lubricates the joints and nourishes the cartilage, further supporting joint health and longevity.

Incorporating Muscle Stretching into Daily Life

Here are four chair yoga exercises designed to improve muscle stretching:

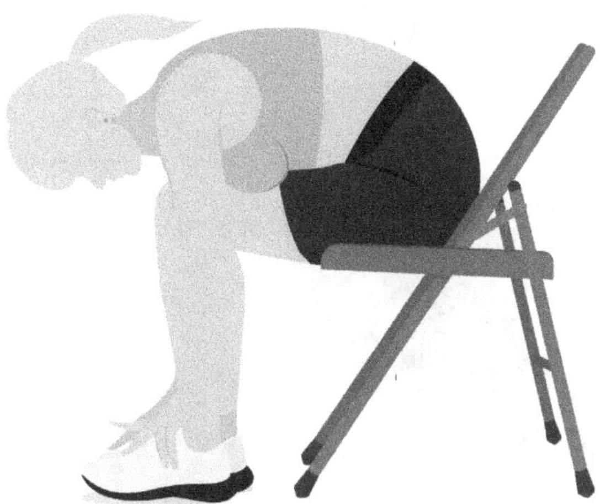

The seated forward bend is a classic yoga pose that provides a deep stretch for the hamstrings, lower back, and calves. By hinging forward at the hips and reaching for the toes, this exercise helps to lengthen and release tension in the back of the legs and spine, promoting better flexibility and mobility. The seated forward bend is also a great way to calm the mind and relieve stress and anxiety, as it encourages deep breathing and a sense of relaxation and release.

Here's how to do it:

1. Sit upright in your chair, ensuring your feet are flat on the ground and your hands are resting on your thighs.
2. While inhaling, straighten your spine and raise your arms above your head.
3. On your exhale, bend forward from your hips, extending your hands towards your feet. Maintain a straight back and an engaged core, and advance only to a point that remains comfortable.
4. Maintain this stretch for 3-5 breaths, concentrating on deep breathing and easing into the stretch.
5. To come out of the stretch, inhale and gradually return to a seated position, aligning your spine one vertebra at a time.

Tips:

- Ensure your back stays straight and your core remains engaged during the stretch to avoid any arching in your spine.
- Proceed only as far as is comfortable, and avoid pushing yourself to reach further towards your toes.
- If you have any lower back pain or injuries, move cautiously and avoid any positions that cause discomfort.

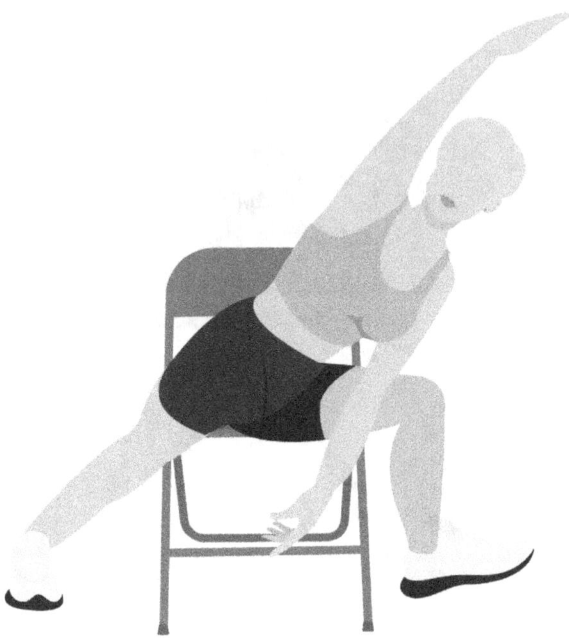

The seated triangle pose is a powerful stretch that targets the sides of the body, including the obliques, intercostals, and shoulders. Extending one arm up towards the ceiling and leaning to the opposite side helps open up the chest and improve posture while also providing a deep stretch for the lateral muscles of the torso. The seated triangle pose can also help to stimulate digestion and improve overall circulation, making it a great choice for seniors looking to maintain optimal health and wellness.

Here's how to do it:

1. Sit straight and tall in your chair, ensuring your feet are firmly planted on the floor.
2. Lift your right arm towards the ceiling, then bend to the left, stretching your right arm over your head.
3. Place your left hand on your left thigh or the chair seat for stability.
4. Keep your chest open and shoulders relaxed, making sure your right shoulder doesn't creep up toward your ear.
5. Maintain this stretch for 3-5 breaths, concentrating on deep, relaxing breaths.
6. To exit the stretch, inhale and smoothly return to a seated position.
7. Switch sides, raising your left arm and leaning to the right, and hold for another 3-5 breaths before gently releasing.

Tips:

- Throughout the stretch, ensure your chest remains open, and your shoulders stay loose, avoiding any scrunching up of your upper body.
- Aim to elongate your spine and take deep breaths into your abdomen as you stretch.
- If you have any neck or shoulder pain or injuries, move cautiously and avoid any positions that cause discomfort.

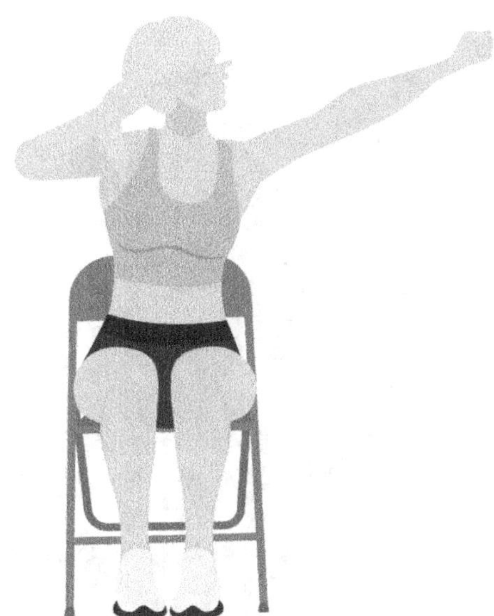

The Bow and Arrow Pose offers several benefits for seniors practicing chair yoga. By mimicking the action of shooting a bow and arrow, this pose helps to strengthen the muscles in the shoulders, arms, and upper back, which can improve overall upper body strength and stability. Additionally, the alternating arm movements help to increase mobility in the shoulders and neck, reducing stiffness and promoting a greater range of motion.

INSTRUCTIONS:

1. Start by sitting straight in your chair, keeping your feet flat on the floor and your spine aligned. Take a moment to relax your shoulders and position your head so it's aligned with your spine.
2. Raise your right arm in front of you at a 45-degree angle, as if you were holding up a bow. Your right hand should be clenched into a fist, with your palm facing downward. Position your arm so that it is in front of the corner of your right eye and slightly above eye level.
3. Next, raise your left arm, also with your palm clenched into a fist, and bring it towards your right arm. Your left arm should be positioned such that both arms are on the right side of your body and parallel to each other.
4. Perform a pulling action with your left arm as if you were drawing back the string of a bow to shoot an arrow. As you pull your left arm back, focus on engaging the muscles in your shoulders, upper back, and arms.
5. Inhale deeply as you pull your left arm back, and then exhale as you release the pulling action, bringing your left arm forward to meet your right arm. Both arms should now be stretched out in front of you.
6. Repeat this push-pull action several times, inhaling as you pull back and exhaling as you release. Aim for 5-10 repetitions or as many as you comfortably can.
7. Once you have completed the desired number of repetitions, return to an upright seated position with both arms resting at your sides.
8. Repeat the entire sequence on the left side, raising your left arm as the "bow" and using your right arm to perform the pulling action.

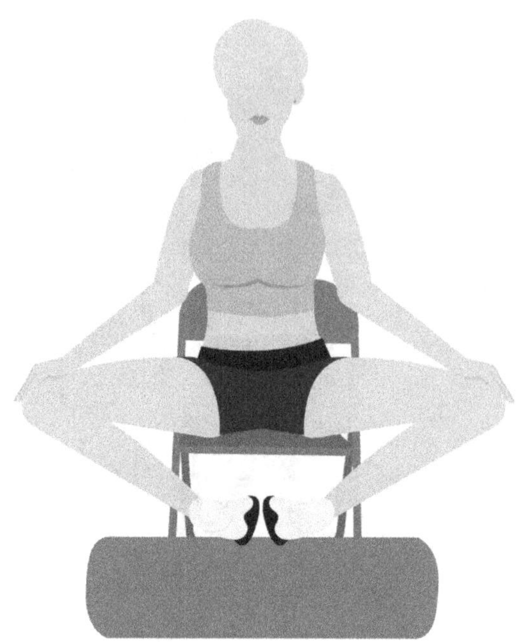

The sitting bound angle posture is a mild hip opener that helps increase flexibility and relieve tension in the hips as well as the inner thighs. This exercise aids in the relaxation and stretching of the muscles as well as connective tissue in the inner thighs and groin, improving hip mobility and range of motion. It does this by drawing the soles of the feet together and letting the knees drop out to the sides. The seated bound angle pose is also a great way to stimulate digestion and improve circulation in the abdominal region, making it a valuable addition to any senior's wellness routine.

Here's how to do it:

1. Your feet should be flat on the ground when you sit up straight in your seat.
2. Bring your feet together, allowing your knees to fall out to the sides.
3. You can get support from blocks or cushions beneath your knees if your hips are too tight.
4. Feel the strain in your groin and inner thighs as you slowly lower your knees to the floor.
5. For three to five breaths, hold the pose, paying close attention to your breathing and letting go of tension.
6. To relieve the strain, gently raise your knees and return your feet to the floor.

Tips:

- Throughout the stretch, maintain a straight back and a tight core to prevent your spine from sagging or rounding.
- Only go as far as feels comfortable for you, and never force or strain to bring your knees down.
- If you have any hip pain or injuries, move cautiously and avoid any positions that cause discomfort.

CHAPTER 11
POSITIONS FOR IMPROVING BALANCE AND STABILITY

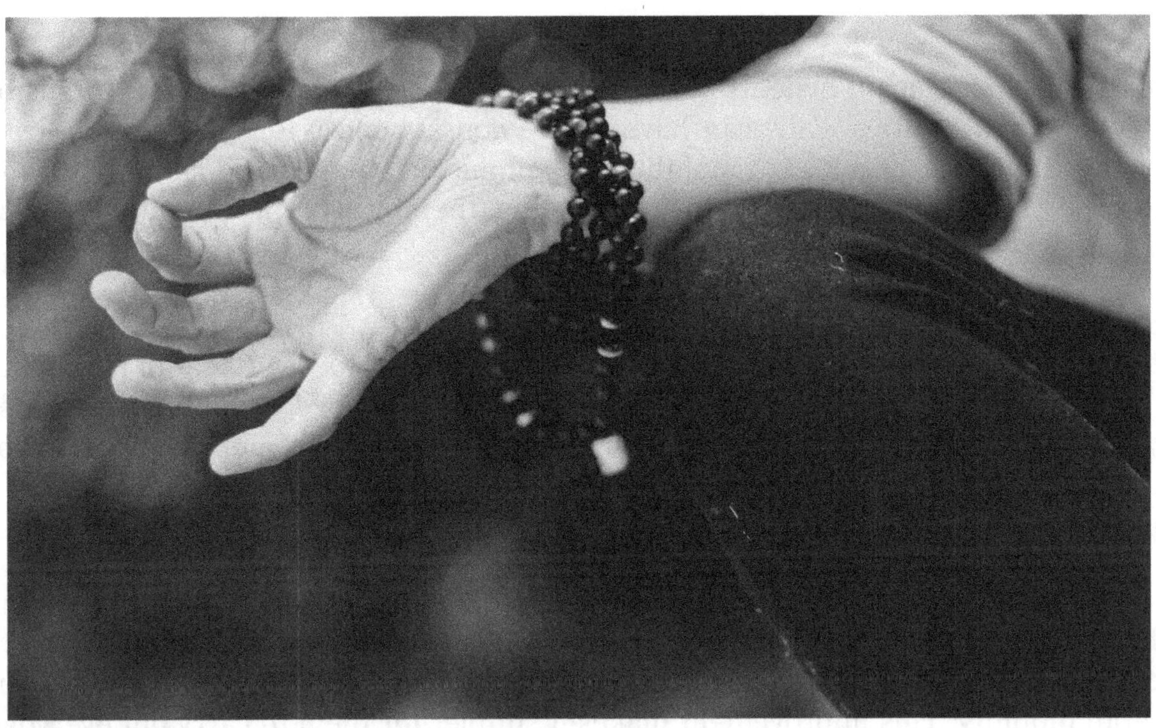

"Balance is not something you find, it's something you create."
- Jana Kingsford

As individuals age, their bodies naturally undergo several changes that can impact their balance and stability. Understanding why enhancing balance and stability is crucial for seniors involves recognizing the specific challenges they face and the potential benefits that come with addressing them.

Firstly, decreased muscle strength and flexibility are common occurrences as people age. Muscles tend to weaken and become less flexible over time, which can affect their ability to support the body and maintain stability. This decline in muscle function contributes to difficulties in performing everyday tasks and increases the risk of falls and injuries.

Moreover, changes in vision and inner ear function can further compromise balance and stability in seniors. Vision is crucial for maintaining balance as it offers spatial awareness and aids in navigating through different environments. As eyesight deteriorates with age, seniors may experience difficulties judging distances and identifying obstacles, making them more susceptible to falls.

Similarly, alterations in inner ear function, which is responsible for detecting motion and maintaining equilibrium, can disrupt the body's balance system. Inner ear issues, such as vestibular disorders or age-related changes in the vestibular system, can lead to dizziness, vertigo, and instability, exacerbating the risk of falls among seniors.

Consequently, seniors face increased risks of falls and injuries due to compromised balance, highlighting the importance of focusing on exercises and activities that promote balance and stability. By proactively tackling these challenges, seniors can reduce the risk of falls and preserve their independence and quality of life as they age.

Now, let's explore the importance of improving balance and stability for seniors and how it helps them in their daily lives:

Importance of Improving Balance and Stability

Preventing Falls and Injuries

One of the most significant benefits of improving balance and stability for seniors is the prevention of falls and injuries. Falls can have severe consequences for older adults, leading to fractures, head injuries, and loss of mobility. By enhancing balance and stability through targeted exercises, seniors can reduce their risk of falling, thereby avoiding potentially life-altering injuries.

Maintaining Independence

Maintaining independence is a top priority for many seniors. However, fear of falling can often limit their mobility and activities, leading to a loss of independence. By improving balance and stability, seniors can regain confidence in their ability to move safely, allowing them to continue performing daily tasks without assistance.

Enhancing Mobility

Good balance and stability are essential for maintaining mobility and agility. As seniors grow older, they often face reductions in muscle strength and flexibility, which can hinder their ability to move freely. Integrating balance and stability exercises into their daily routines can enhance their overall mobility. This improvement makes it simpler for them to carry out everyday tasks such as walking, climbing stairs, and rising from or sitting in chairs.

Boosting Confidence

A strong sense of confidence is crucial for seniors to remain active and engaged in life. Improving balance and stability can boost confidence levels by providing seniors with the reassurance that they can navigate their environment safely. This increased confidence encourages them to participate in social activities, exercise classes, and outings without the fear of falling or getting injured.

Improving Posture

Maintaining good posture becomes increasingly challenging as we age, primarily due to changes in muscle strength and flexibility. Poor posture has a negative impact on balance and stability, as well as causing discomfort and suffering. Seniors can improve their posture by integrating balance and stability exercises, which lowers their risk of back discomfort and other musculoskeletal ailments.

Enhancing Cognitive Function

There is growing evidence to suggest that physical activity, including balance and stability exercises, can have a positive impact on cognitive function in seniors. By engaging in activities that challenge balance and coordination, seniors can stimulate brain function and improve cognitive skills such as memory and attention.

Ultimately, enhancing balance and stability can greatly improve the overall quality of life for seniors. By reducing the risk of falls and injuries, maintaining independence, and increasing confidence and mobility, seniors can enjoy a higher level of well-being and satisfaction in their later years.

How Can Yoga Contribute to Maintaining Stability

Yoga emerges as a gentle yet powerful tool for seniors seeking to bolster their stability and balance. Through its emphasis on deliberate movements, breath awareness, and mindful poses, yoga presents a myriad of benefits for older adults endeavoring to enhance their physical well-being. Within the serene confines of a yoga studio or the comfort of their own homes, seniors can embark on a transformative journey towards improved stability and balance.

At the core of yoga's efficacy lies its ability to strengthen the body's central support system—the core muscles. Yoga poses, ranging from gentle stretches to more challenging balances, engage muscles of the abdomen, obliques, and lower back. This focus on core strength not only fortifies the spine but also serves as a cornerstone for maintaining stability and preventing falls, crucial concerns for seniors navigating their daily lives.

Furthermore, yoga serves as a gateway to enhanced flexibility—a quality often compromised with age. Through a series of gentle stretches and lengthening movements, yoga fosters greater flexibility in muscles, tendons, and ligaments. This new-found suppleness not only facilitates ease of movement but also reduces the risk of injury, laying the groundwork for improved balance and stability.

Proprioception, the body's innate ability to perceive its position in space, receives ample attention in the practice of yoga. Balancing poses and coordinated movements challenge seniors to develop heightened proprioceptive awareness, enabling them to better control their movements and maintain stability—skills that prove invaluable in navigating everyday activities with confidence and grace.

Mindfulness lies at the heart of the yoga experience, offering seniors a pathway to greater presence and awareness. Through focused attention on breath and bodily sensations, seniors cultivate mindfulness both on and off the yoga mat. This heightened awareness translates into improved concentration, sharper focus, and ultimately, better balance and stability in their daily endeavors.

Standing poses emerge as pillars of strength in the yoga practice for seniors. Postures like Mountain Pose, Warrior Pose, and Tree Pose challenge individuals to ground themselves firmly through their feet, distributing weight evenly and strengthening muscles of the legs and ankles. With each steady breath and deliberate movement, seniors inch closer to a state of equilibrium and poise.

Yoga props, such as blocks, straps, and chairs, serve as invaluable aids for seniors navigating balance and mobility challenges. These supportive tools provide stability and assistance, allowing seniors to modify poses and gradually build strength and confidence without risking injury or strain.

Incorporating balance challenges into yoga practice further hones seniors' strength, coordination, and confidence. From standing on one leg to transitioning between poses fluidly, these challenges foster resilience and fortitude, paving the way for improved balance and stability in both body and mind.

Attention to alignment emerges as a guiding principle in yoga practice, ensuring seniors maintain stability and balance in each pose. By aligning their bodies correctly and engaging the appropriate muscles for support, seniors cultivate a sense of symmetry and strength that transcends the confines of the yoga mat.

Finally, relaxation techniques, such as deep breathing, guided meditation, and Corpse Pose, serve as the culmination of the yoga practice. By releasing tension and quieting the mind, seniors create a space for profound relaxation and rejuvenation, nurturing a body-mind connection that fosters stability and balance in their daily lives.

In summary, yoga stands as a beacon of hope and healing for seniors seeking to enhance their stability and balance. Through its holistic approach to physical and mental well-being, yoga empowers seniors to strengthen their core, improve flexibility, heighten proprioceptive awareness, and cultivate mindfulness—all of which contribute to a life of stability, balance, and vitality.

How to Improve Balance and Stability

Whether you're a senior looking to maintain independence or an athlete aiming to enhance performance, incorporating specific positions and exercises into your routine can significantly improve balance and stability. These positions target various muscle groups, enhance proprioception (the body's awareness of its position in space), and promote overall coordination. Let's explore some key positions and exercises that can help improve balance and stability:

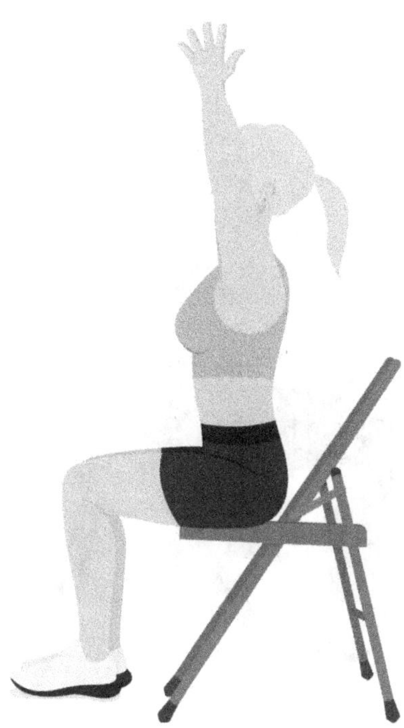

The seated mountain pose is a foundational posture that promotes good posture, balance, and stability. This exercise engages your core muscles, strengthens your spine, and improves your overall body awareness. By concentrating on your breathing and keeping a steady, upright posture, you can lessen stress and boost your feelings of calmness and stability. Here's how to go about it:

1. Keep your back straight, feet flat on the floor, and hands on thighs as you sit tall in your chair.
2. Envision a thread running from your head to the tip of your spine, drawing you up and out of your body.
3. Keep your shoulders down and relaxed while you contract your core muscles to elevate your chest.
4. Breathe deeply a few times, paying attention to your posture and balance.

Tips for Seated Mountain Pose:

- Keep your feet firmly planted on the floor throughout the pose, feeling your connection to the earth.
- Lift your chest and use your core muscles while avoiding slouching or rounding your spine.
- Concentrate on your breath and attempt to remain calm and stable throughout the position.

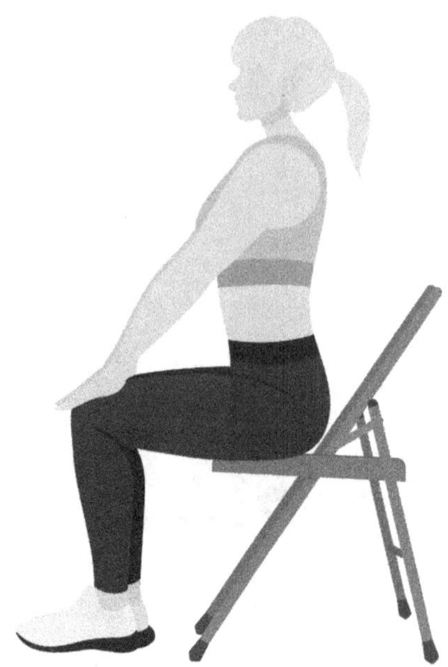

The seated chair pose is an excellent way to strengthen your leg and core muscles, which are essential for maintaining balance and stability. This exercise also helps to improve circulation, increase energy levels, and boost your overall mood. By engaging your core and keeping your feet firmly planted on the floor, you can build a strong foundation for more challenging balance poses.

Here's how to do it:

1. Keep your back straight, feet flat on the floor, and hands on thighs as you sit tall in your chair.
2. Bring your knees up to your chest and move your weight forward so that your hips are off the chair.
3. To keep from wobbling, grab the chair's armrests or, for an extra challenge, spread your arms wide.
4. Avoid slouching or bringing your shoulders down to your ears by keeping your core engaged and your chest raised.
5. Then, after three to five breaths in the posture, slowly bring your hips back down to the chair.

Tips for Seated Chair Pose:

- Keep your feet firmly planted on the floor throughout the pose, feeling your connection to the earth.
- Engage your core muscles and lift your chest, avoiding any slouching or rounding in your spine.
- If you have any knee or hip pain or injuries, move cautiously and avoid any positions that cause discomfort.

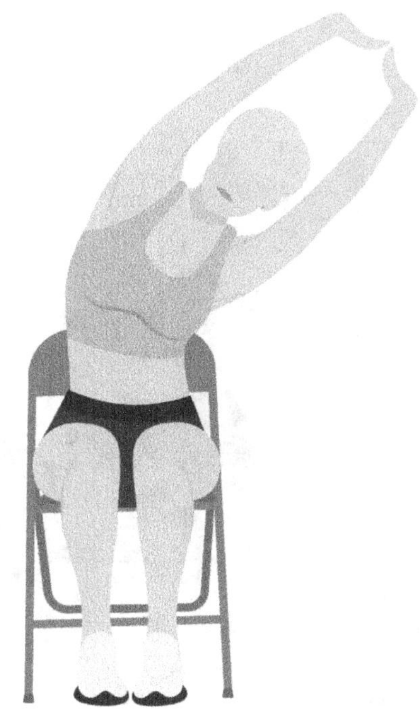

The Crescent Moon Bend, also known as Urdhva Hastasana, is a chair yoga posture that focuses on building flexibility in the ribcage and providing elasticity to the waist. As we age, it is common to experience stiffness or aches in the intercostal muscles and waist area, which can be prevented by regularly practicing side bends like the Crescent Moon Bend. This posture also activates a new movement for the spinal cord, encouraging it to arch into a C-shape, which is believed to improve memory and concentration according to traditional yoga teachings.

Instructions:

1. To start, sit up straight on your chair, feet together and flat on the floor. All the while you're practicing, keep your toes close together.
2. Breathe in deeply (in) and bring your hands up to your chest, palms facing each other. Throughout the workout, keep your arms extended and your shoulders relaxed.
3. Breathe out slowly as you arch your back slightly to the right, creating a crescent shape. Take your time and be careful not to make any sudden moves. If you experience any discomfort, pause and hold the position, focusing on your breath and the sensations in your body. Keep your shoulders spread wide and away from your ears.
4. Hold the Crescent Moon Bend to the right for 3-5 breaths, or as long as comfortable, observing the sensations in your body and allowing your muscles to relax and lengthen with each exhalation.
5. To release the pose, inhale and slowly return to an upright seated position, bringing your arms back down to rest on your knees. Take a moment to relax and observe any changes in your body.
6. Repeat the Crescent Moon Bend on the left side, following the same instructions and holding the pose for an equal number of breaths.

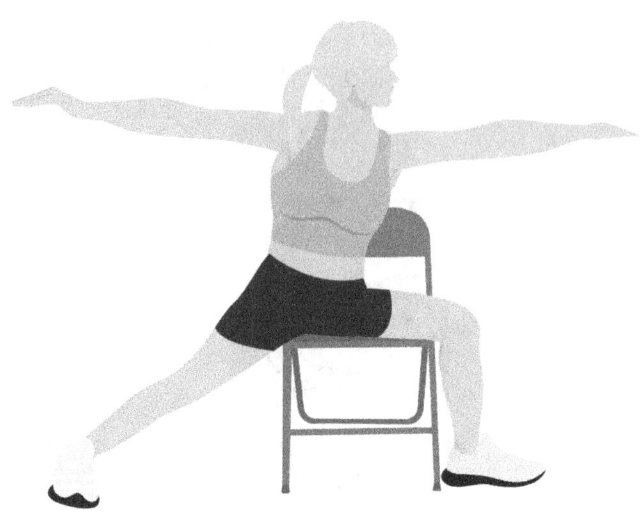

The seated warrior III pose is a more advanced balance posture that strengthens your legs, core, and back muscles. This exercise also helps to improve your focus, concentration, and overall body alignment. By keeping your back straight and your core engaged, you can build strength and stability in your entire body, while also challenging your balance and coordination.

Here's how to do it:

1. Prop your feet firmly on the floor and sit up straight in your chair.
2. Place your weight on your left foot and, while maintaining a straight knee, raise your right leg behind you.
3. With your arms extended wide, bend forward at the hips and lower your body until your torso is parallel to the floor (or as near as you feel comfortable).
4. Maintain a straight back and an engaged core, and avoid allowing your shoulders to slouch up toward your ears.
5. Stay in the position for three to five breaths, paying close attention to your breathing and keeping your balance.
6. Return to a relaxed position by gently raising your upper body and bringing your right leg back down to the floor.
7. Repeat the position on the other side, elevating your left leg and holding for 3-5 breaths before letting go.

Tips for Seated Warrior III:

- Avoid slouching or curving your spine by keeping your back straight and core engaged throughout the position.
- Keeping your eyes on anything stationary in front of you will help you stay balanced.
- If you have any lower back pain or injuries, move cautiously and avoid any positions that cause discomfort.

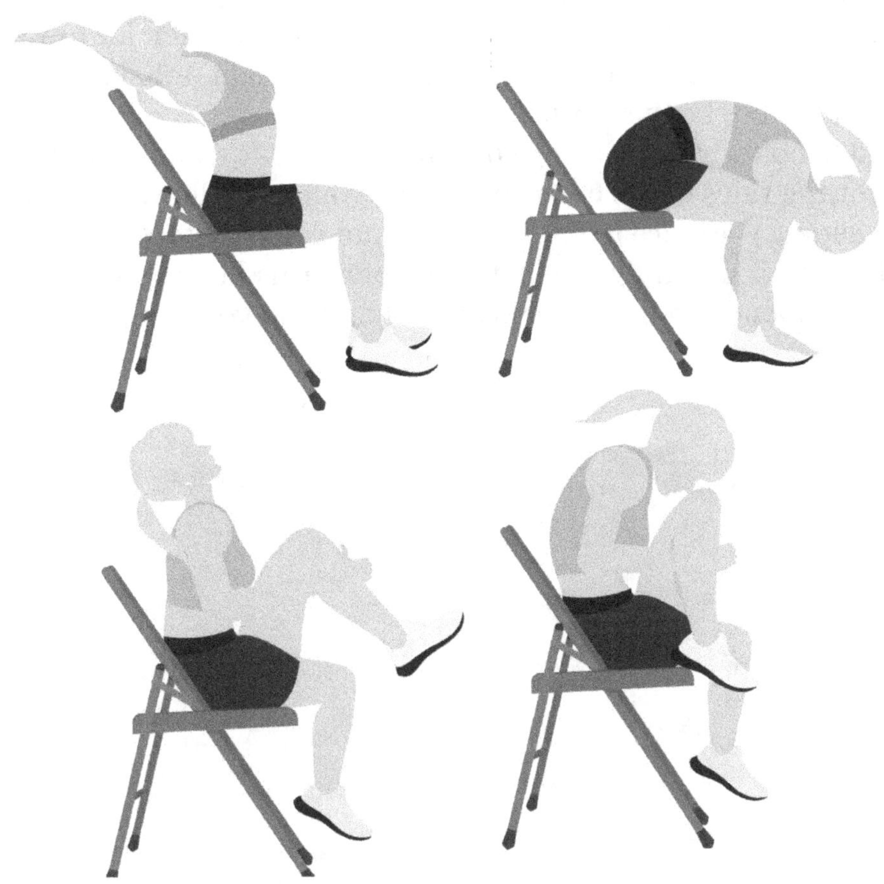

Sun Salutations, or Suryanamaskar, is a revered yoga sequence that combines multiple postures to promote holistic health. This graceful series of movements is designed to maintain body-mind balance, improve blood circulation, stimulate various muscle groups, nerves, and internal organs, and provide grace and tone to the body. The sun is regarded by many cultures as the ultimate source of energy and life, making Sun Salutations a fitting tribute to this vital force. When practicing this posture sequence, it is essential to move through each position without hurry, holding each posture for about six counts before transitioning to the next.

INSTRUCTIONS:

1. Begin in an upright seated position, with your feet hip-width apart to maintain proper weight distribution. Create a prayer position by bringing your hands together and placing them in front of your chest. Breathe in deeply and out slowly, bringing your attention to the breath and the here and now.

2. As you inhale, lift both hands overhead, arching your body back slightly. Hold this position while facing the sky, with your arms pushed back. Be mindful not to push your neck beyond its comfortable range of motion.

3. Exhale as you bend forward, bringing your hands down towards the ground. Aim to touch your fingertips to your toes, but if this is not possible, simply stretch as far as comfortable. Keep your fingertips together and glance forward, maintaining a straight spine.

4. As you breathe in, bring your right leg up to your chest and, using both hands, grasp your hamstring. Lean on the chair with your right foot if you're having trouble keeping your balance. Keep your head and neck in an arched position, looking up at the ceiling, for a few counts.

5. While holding the lunge position, slowly bend your neck to rest your forehead on your right knee, bringing your thigh closer to your chest. Maintain this position for several breaths, then gently return your right leg to the starting position.

6. Exhale and lean forward once more, this time raising your left leg toward your chest. Hold the left leg in the same manner as you did with the right, inhaling and then releasing the left foot back to the starting position.

7. Exhale and bend forward, placing your palms on your shins. Continue bending forward, reaching for the sides of the chair to support yourself. Allow your spine to gently stretch forward, keeping your face looking forward and your neck in line with your spine.

8. Breathe in and sit up straight, extending your arms above your head. Breathe out and settle into the mountain pose, placing your hands on your thighs and keeping your spine aligned.

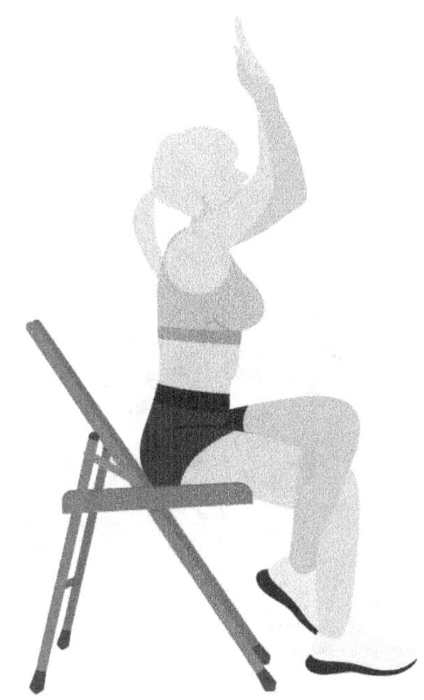

The seated eagle balance pose is a challenging posture that improves balance, coordination, and focus. This exercise also helps to stretch your hips, shoulders, and upper back, while strengthening your core muscles and arms. By crossing your legs and arms in a specific pattern, you create a sense of stability and grounding, making it easier to maintain your balance.

Here's how to do it:

1. Sit upright in your chair, ensuring your feet are firmly planted on the ground.
2. Place your right thigh over your left thigh and, if you can, loop your right foot behind your left calf.
3. Stretch your arms forward, then overlap your left arm over your right, attempting to join your palms together or bring them as close as you can.
4. Elevate your elbows to the level of your shoulders and press your hands together (or the backs of your hands if your palms don't meet).
5. Lift your feet off the ground, balancing on your sitting bones.
6. Maintain this position for 3-5 breaths, concentrating on deep breathing and keeping your balance.
7. To come out of the pose, carefully separate your arms and legs, and place your feet back on the ground.
8. Switch sides and perform the pose again, this time crossing your left thigh over your right and your right arm over your left, holding for another 3-5 breaths before gently releasing the position.

Tips for Seated Eagle Balance:

- Throughout the position, be sure to keep your back straight and core tight. Don't slouch or curve your spine in any way.
- If you can't wrap your foot behind your calf, simply cross your thighs and rest your top foot on your bottom thigh.
- If you have any shoulder or hip pain or injuries, move cautiously and avoid any positions that cause discomfort.

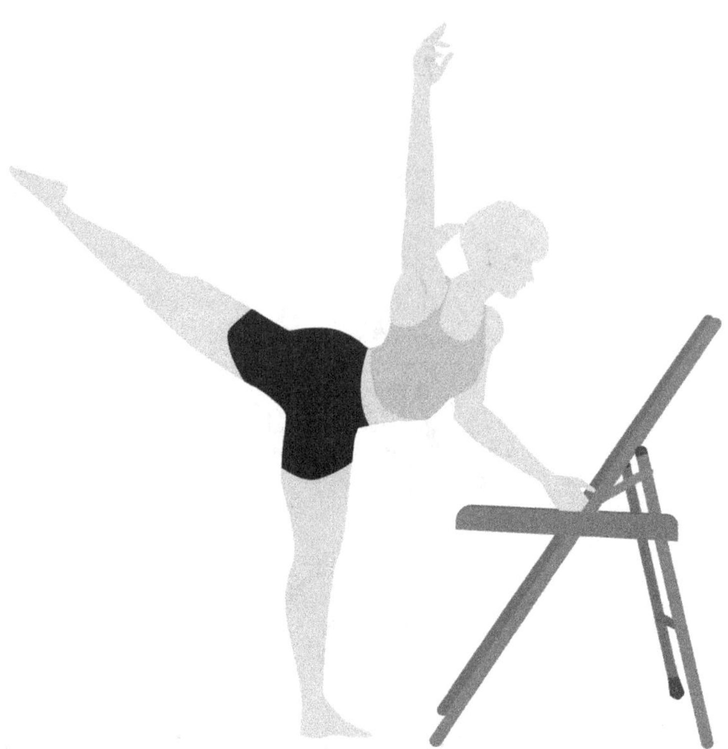

The seated half moon balance pose is an excellent way to challenge your balance and stability while stretching the sides of your body. This exercise helps to strengthen your core muscles and legs, while also improving your focus and concentration. By keeping your chest open and your shoulders relaxed, you can maintain proper alignment and balance throughout the pose.

Here's how to do it:

1. Position yourself in a tall posture, feet flat on the floor.
2. Place your right foot firmly on the left sit bone and stretch your right leg to the side.
3. Lean to the left and extend your right arm above your head while reaching up toward the ceiling with your right arm.
4. To steady yourself, put your left hand on your left leg or the chair's seat.
5. Refrain from hunching your right shoulder towards your ear and maintain an open chest and loose shoulders.
6. Stay in the position for three to five breaths, paying close attention to your breathing and keeping your balance.
7. To come out of the posture, gently bring your right leg back down to the floor while raising your chest back up.
8. Repeat the posture on the opposite side, rising your left leg and stretching your left arm up and over. Hold for 3-5 breaths before releasing.

Tips for Seated Half-Moon Balance:

- Keep your chest open and your shoulders relaxed throughout the pose, avoiding any hunching or tension in your upper body.
- Focus on lengthening your spine and breathing deeply into your belly throughout the pose.
- If you have any neck or shoulder pain or injuries, move cautiously and avoid any positions that cause discomfort.

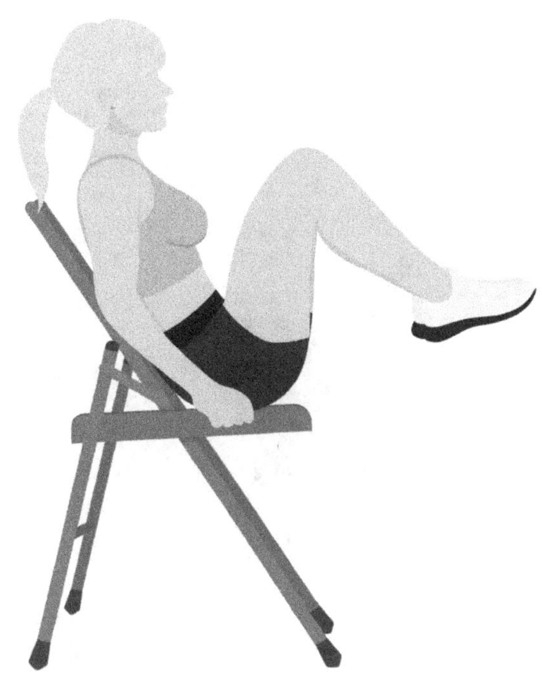

The seated boat pose is a powerful core-strengthening exercise that also improves balance and stability. This pose engages your abdominal muscles, lower back, and hip flexors, helping to create a strong and stable foundation for your body. Additionally, the seated boat pose stimulates your digestive system and improves overall digestion.

Here's how to do it:

1. Ensure proper posture by sitting upright in your chair, with your feet firmly planted on the floor and your hands calmly resting on your thighs.
2. Elevate your feet, aligning your shins with the floor (or as close as is comfortable for you).
3. Extend your arms forward, maintaining a relaxed and lowered shoulder position.
4. Maintain proper posture by keeping your back straight and engaging your core. Be mindful of avoiding any rounding of your lower back or hunching of your shoulders towards your ears.
5. Maintain your balance and take deep breaths while holding the stance for three to five minutes.
6. When you're ready to end the pose, carefully bring your feet down to the ground and place your hands on your thighs.

Tips for Seated Boat Pose:

- Maintain proper posture and engage your core during the pose to prevent any curvature or slouching in your back.
- If you have any lower back pain or injuries, move cautiously and avoid any positions that cause discomfort.
- You can modify the pose by keeping your knees bent and your feet on the floor, or by holding onto the sides of the chair for support.

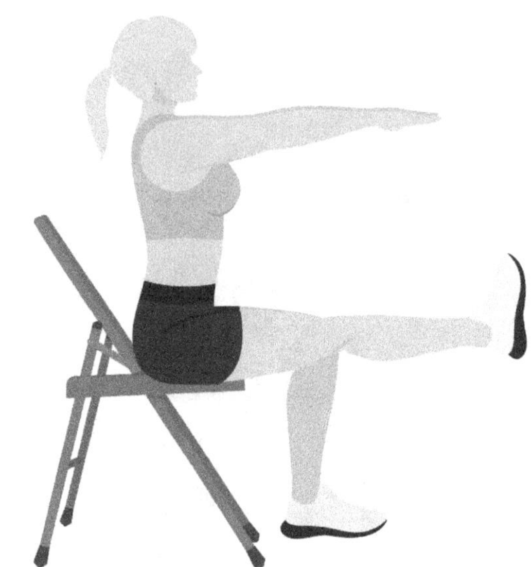

The seated single-leg balance pose is an excellent way to challenge your balance and stability while strengthening your legs and core muscles. This exercise helps to improve your focus, concentration, and overall body awareness. By keeping your back straight and your core engaged, you can maintain proper alignment and balance throughout the pose, promoting better posture and reducing the risk of falls.

Here's how to do it:

1. Position your hands on your thighs and sit up straight in your chair with your feet flat on the floor.
2. Raise your right foot off the floor and extend your leg forward, reaching as far as you can without any discomfort.
3. Avoid allowing your hips or shoulders to move or rotate. Instead, maintain a straight back and a tight core.
4. Uphold the pose for 3-5 breaths, emphasizing deep breathing and balance.
5. To finish the pose, carefully bring your right foot down to the ground.
6. Repeat the pose on the other side, lifting your left leg and holding for 3-5 breaths before releasing.

Tips for Seated Single-Leg Balance:

- Aim to prevent slouching or curving your spine by maintaining a straight back and a tight core throughout the position.
- To assist you in staying balanced, concentrate your eyes on a stationary spot in front of you.
- If you have any knee or hip pain or injuries, move cautiously and avoid any positions that cause discomfort.

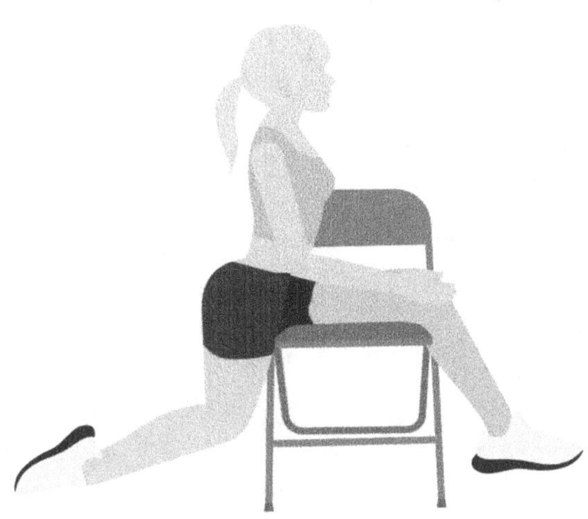

The seated dancer's pose is a beautiful and challenging balance posture that improves balance, flexibility, and stability. This exercise strengthens your legs, core, and back muscles, while also opening your chest and shoulders. To enhance your general body awareness and alleviate stress and anxiety, it is beneficial to concentrate on your breath and maintain a solid and upright posture.

This is how you do it:

1. Sit straight in your chair with your feet firmly planted on the ground and your hands resting on your thighs.
2. Shift your weight to your left sitting bone and raise your right leg behind you, bending at the knee. Reach back with your right hand to hold your right foot or ankle.
3. Gently push your right foot against your hand, lifting your leg upward and backward. Extend your left arm forward and upward, inducing a mild arch in your back.
4. Keep your chest raised and your core tight, ensuring your shoulders don't creep up towards your ears.
5. Hold this position for 3-5 breaths, concentrating on deep breathing and stability. To exit the pose, slowly lower your right leg to the ground and place your hands back on your thighs.
6. Repeat the pose on the other side, lifting your left leg and reaching back with your left hand, holding for 3-5 breaths before releasing.

Tips for Seated Dancer's Pose:

- Keep your chest lifted and your core engaged throughout the pose, avoiding any slouching or rounding in your spine.
- If you can't reach your foot or ankle, you can use a strap or towel to help extend your reach.
- If you have any lower back pain or injuries, move cautiously and avoid any positions that cause discomfort.

By integrating these ten balance and stability exercises into your chair yoga routine, you can enhance your overall balance, coordination, and stability. This will lower the chances of experiencing falls or injuries and ultimately enhance your quality of life. Always remember to approach your practice with a professional mindset, taking the time to move slowly and mindfully. It's important to listen to your body and make any necessary modifications to the poses to ensure they align with your individual needs and abilities. Through consistent dedication and perseverance, one can cultivate enhanced physical prowess, adaptability, and self-assurance.

CHAPTER 12

DAY-BY-DAY COMPREHENSIVE POSE PROGRAM TO TONE, STABILIZE AND LOSE WEIGHT

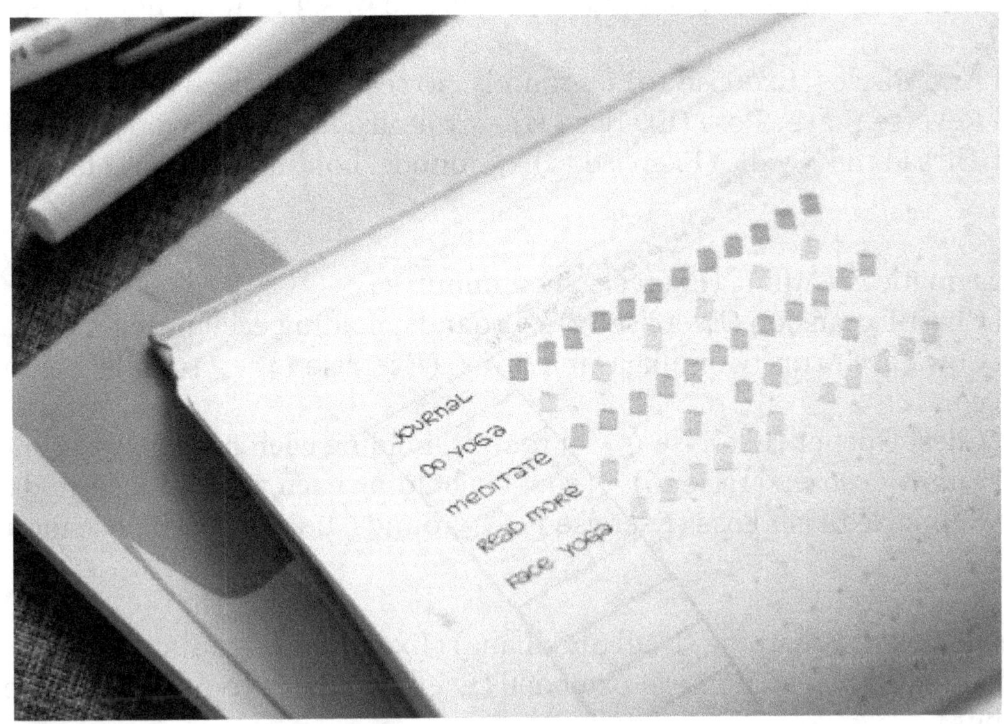

While yoga might not be the most vigorous exercise, its effectiveness for toning and shedding pounds shouldn't be overlooked.

This chapter provides a sample day-by-day yoga program designed to target different muscle groups, strengthen your core, enhance stability, and promote weight loss. Remember, consistency is key. By incorporating this routine into your lifestyle and maintaining a healthy diet, you can experience the transformative power of yoga on your physical and mental well-being.

Sample Day-by-Day Yoga Program

Day 1:
- Diaphragmatic Breathing (Exercise 1) - 2 minutes
- Alternate Nostril Breathing (Nadi Shodhana) (Exercise 2) - 2 minutes
- Starting Position (Chapter 8) - 1 minute
- Circles to Start Warm Up (Exercise 3) - 2 minutes
- See-Saw Feet Warm Up (Exercise 4) - 2 minutes
- Seated Cat-Cow (Exercise 5) - 3 rounds, holding each pose for 4 seconds
- Seated Torso Twists (Exercise 6) - 3 rounds, holding each pose for 4 seconds

Day 2:
- Alternate Nostril Breathing (Nadi Shodhana) (Exercise 2) - 2 minutes
- The Lazy Stretch Warm-Up (Exercise 7) - 2 minutes
- Seated Shoulder Rolls (Exercise 8) - 2 rounds, 30 seconds in each direction
- Seated Eagle Arms (Garudasana Arms) (Exercise 9) - 3 rounds, holding each pose for 4 seconds
- Seated Arm Circles (Exercise 10) - 2 rounds, 30 seconds in each direction
- Seated Reverse Prayer Pose (Exercise 11) - 3 rounds, holding each pose for 4 seconds
- Seated Thread the Needle (Exercise 12) - 3 rounds, holding each pose for 4 seconds

Day 3:
- Diaphragmatic Breathing (Exercise 1) - 2 minutes
- Seated Chest Expansion (Exercise 13) - 3 rounds, holding each pose for 4 seconds
- Seated Cow Face Arms (Gomukhasana Arms) (Exercise 14) - 3 rounds, holding each pose for 4 seconds
- Seated Chest Opener (Exercise 15) - 3 rounds, holding each pose for 4 seconds
- Seated Puppy Pose (Exercise 16) - 3 rounds, holding each pose for 4 seconds
- Seated Supported Fish Pose (Exercise 17) - 3 rounds, holding each pose for 4 seconds

Day 4:
- Alternate Nostril Breathing (Nadi Shodhana) (Exercise 2) - 2 minutes
- Seated Forward Bend with Legs Extended (Exercise 18) - 3 rounds, holding each pose for 4 seconds
- Seated Pigeon Pose (Exercise 19) - 3 rounds, holding each pose for 4 seconds
- Seated Tree Pose (Exercise 20) - 3 rounds, holding each pose for 4 seconds
- Seated Hamstring Stretch (Exercise 21) - 3 rounds, holding each pose for 4 seconds
- Hero's Pose (Exercise 22) - 3 rounds, holding each pose for 4 seconds

Day 5:
- Diaphragmatic Breathing (Exercise 1) - 2 minutes
- Seated Foot and Ankle Rolls (Exercise 23) - 2 rounds, 30 seconds in each direction
- Seated Leg Lifts (Exercise 24) - 3 rounds, holding each pose for 4 seconds
- Seated Knee to Chest (Exercise 25) - 3 rounds, holding each pose for 4 seconds
- Seated Calf Raises (Exercise 26) - 3 rounds, holding each pose for 4 seconds
- Seated Toe Taps (Exercise 27) - 2 rounds, 30 seconds each round

Day 6:
- Alternate Nostril Breathing (Nadi Shodhana) (Exercise 2) - 2 minutes
- Seated Leg Extensions (Exercise 28) - 3 rounds, holding each pose for 4 seconds
- Seated Leg Circles (Exercise 29) - 2 rounds, 30 seconds in each direction
- Chair Yoga Lunge Pose (Exercise 30) - 3 rounds, holding each pose for 4 seconds
- Half Supine Pose (Exercise 31) - 3 rounds, holding each pose for 4 seconds
- Seated Eagle Legs (Exercise 32) - 3 rounds, holding each pose for 4 seconds

Day 7:
- Diaphragmatic Breathing (Exercise 1) - 2 minutes
- Side Angle Pose (Exercise 33) - 3 rounds, holding each pose for 4 seconds
- Child's Pose (Exercise 34) - 3 rounds, holding each pose for 4 seconds
- Seated Figure-4 Stretch (Exercise 35) - 3 rounds, holding each pose for 4 seconds
- Seated Butterfly Pose (Exercise 36) - 3 rounds, holding each pose for 4 seconds

Day 8:
- Alternate Nostril Breathing (Nadi Shodhana) (Exercise 2) - 2 minutes
- Seated Forward Bend (Exercise 37) - 3 rounds, holding each pose for 4 seconds
- Seated Triangle Pose (Exercise 38) - 3 rounds, holding each pose for 4 seconds
- Bow and Arrow Pose (Exercise 39) - 3 rounds, holding each pose for 4 seconds
- Seated Bound Angle Pose (Exercise 40) - 3 rounds, holding each pose for 4 seconds

Day 9:
- Diaphragmatic Breathing (Exercise 1) - 2 minutes
- Seated Mountain Pose (Exercise 41) - 3 rounds, holding each pose for 4 seconds
- Seated Chair Pose (Exercise 42) - 3 rounds, holding each pose for 4 seconds
- Crescent Moon Bend (Exercise 43) - 3 rounds, holding each pose for 4 seconds
- Seated Warrior III (Exercise 44) - 3 rounds, holding each pose for 4 seconds

Day 10:
- Alternate Nostril Breathing (Nadi Shodhana) (Exercise 2) - 2 minutes
- Sun Salutations (Exercise 45) - 3 rounds, holding each pose for 4 seconds
- Seated Eagle Balance (Exercise 46) - 3 rounds, holding each pose for 4 seconds
- Seated Half Moon Balance (Exercise 47) - 3 rounds, holding each pose for 4 seconds
- Seated Boat Pose (Exercise 48) - 3 rounds, holding each pose for 4 seconds

Day 11:
- Diaphragmatic Breathing (Exercise 1) - 2 minutes
- Seated Single-Leg Balance (Exercise 49) - 3 rounds, holding each pose for 4 seconds
- Seated Dancer's Pose (Exercise 50) - 3 rounds, holding each pose for 4 seconds
- Circles to Start Warm Up (Exercise 3) - 2 minutes
- See-Saw Feet Warm Up (Exercise 4) - 2 minutes
- Seated Cat-Cow (Exercise 5) - 3 rounds, holding each pose for 4 seconds
- Seated Torso Twists (Exercise 6) - 3 rounds, holding each pose for 4 seconds

Day 12:
- Alternate Nostril Breathing (Nadi Shodhana) (Exercise 2) - 2 minutes
- The Lazy Stretch Warm-Up (Exercise 7) - 2 minutes
- Seated Shoulder Rolls (Exercise 8) - 2 rounds, 30 seconds in each direction
- Seated Eagle Arms (Garudasana Arms) (Exercise 9) - 3 rounds, holding each pose for 4 seconds
- Seated Arm Circles (Exercise 10) - 2 rounds, 30 seconds in each direction
- Seated Reverse Prayer Pose (Exercise 11) - 3 rounds, holding each pose for 4 seconds
- Seated Thread the Needle (Exercise 12) - 3 rounds, holding each pose for 4 seconds

Day 13:
- Diaphragmatic Breathing (Exercise 1) - 2 minutes
- Seated Chest Expansion (Exercise 13) - 3 rounds, holding each pose for 4 seconds
- Seated Cow Face Arms (Gomukhasana Arms) (Exercise 14) - 3 rounds, holding each pose for 4 seconds
- Seated Chest Opener (Exercise 15) - 3 rounds, holding each pose for 4 seconds
- Seated Puppy Pose (Exercise 16) - 3 rounds, holding each pose for 4 seconds
- Seated Supported Fish Pose (Exercise 17) - 3 rounds, holding each pose for 4 seconds

Day 14:
- Alternate Nostril Breathing (Nadi Shodhana) (Exercise 2) - 2 minutes
- Seated Forward Bend with Legs Extended (Exercise 18) - 3 rounds, holding each pose for 4 seconds
- Seated Pigeon Pose (Exercise 19) - 3 rounds, holding each pose for 4 seconds
- Seated Tree Pose (Exercise 20) - 3 rounds, holding each pose for 4 seconds
- Seated Hamstring Stretch (Exercise 21) - 3 rounds, holding each pose for 4 seconds
- Hero's Pose (Exercise 22) - 3 rounds, holding each pose for 4 seconds

Day 15:
- Diaphragmatic Breathing (Exercise 1) - 2 minutes
- Seated Foot and Ankle Rolls (Exercise 23) - 2 rounds, 30 seconds in each direction
- Seated Leg Lifts (Exercise 24) - 3 rounds, holding each pose for 4 seconds
- Seated Knee to Chest (Exercise 25) - 3 rounds, holding each pose for 4 seconds
- Seated Calf Raises (Exercise 26) - 3 rounds, holding each pose for 4 seconds
- Seated Toe Taps (Exercise 27) - 2 rounds, 30 seconds each round

Day 16:
- Alternate Nostril Breathing (Nadi Shodhana) (Exercise 2) - 2 minutes
- Seated Leg Extensions (Exercise 28) - 3 rounds, holding each pose for 4 seconds
- Seated Leg Circles (Exercise 29) - 2 rounds, 30 seconds in each direction
- Chair Yoga Lunge Pose (Exercise 30) - 3 rounds, holding each pose for 4 seconds
- Half Supine Pose (Exercise 31) - 3 rounds, holding each pose for 4 seconds
- Seated Eagle Legs (Exercise 32) - 3 rounds, holding each pose for 4 seconds

Day 17:
- Diaphragmatic Breathing (Exercise 1) - 2 minutes
- Side Angle Pose (Exercise 33) - 3 rounds, holding each pose for 4 seconds
- Child's Pose (Exercise 34) - 3 rounds, holding each pose for 4 seconds
- Seated Figure-4 Stretch (Exercise 35) - 3 rounds, holding each pose for 4 seconds
- Seated Butterfly Pose (Exercise 36) - 3 rounds, holding each pose for 4 seconds

Day 18:
- Alternate Nostril Breathing (Nadi Shodhana) (Exercise 2) - 2 minutes
- Seated Forward Bend (Exercise 37) - 3 rounds, holding each pose for 4 seconds
- Seated Triangle Pose (Exercise 38) - 3 rounds, holding each pose for 4 seconds
- Bow and Arrow Pose (Exercise 39) - 3 rounds, holding each pose for 4 seconds
- Seated Bound Angle Pose (Exercise 40) - 3 rounds, holding each pose for 4 seconds

Day 19:
- Diaphragmatic Breathing (Exercise 1) - 2 minutes
- Seated Mountain Pose (Exercise 41) - 3 rounds, holding each pose for 4 seconds
- Seated Chair Pose (Exercise 42) - 3 rounds, holding each pose for 4 seconds
- Crescent Moon Bend (Exercise 43) - 3 rounds, holding each pose for 4 seconds
- Seated Warrior III (Exercise 44) - 3 rounds, holding each pose for 4 seconds

Day 20:
- Alternate Nostril Breathing (Nadi Shodhana) (Exercise 2) - 2 minutes
- Sun Salutations (Exercise 45) - 3 rounds, holding each pose for 4 seconds
- Seated Eagle Balance (Exercise 46) - 3 rounds, holding each pose for 4 seconds
- Seated Half Moon Balance (Exercise 47) - 3 rounds, holding each pose for 4 seconds
- Seated Boat Pose (Exercise 48) - 3 rounds, holding each pose for 4 seconds

Day 21:
- Diaphragmatic Breathing (Exercise 1) - 2 minutes
- Seated Single-Leg Balance (Exercise 49) - 3 rounds, holding each pose for 4 seconds
- Seated Dancer's Pose (Exercise 50) - 3 rounds, holding each pose for 4 seconds
- Circles to Start Warm Up (Exercise 3) - 2 minutes
- See-Saw Feet Warm Up (Exercise 4) - 2 minutes
- Seated Cat-Cow (Exercise 5) - 3 rounds, holding each pose for 4 seconds
- Seated Torso Twists (Exercise 6) - 3 rounds, holding each pose for 4 seconds

Day 22:
- Alternate Nostril Breathing (Nadi Shodhana) (Exercise 2) - 2 minutes
- The Lazy Stretch Warm-Up (Exercise 7) - 2 minutes
- Seated Shoulder Rolls (Exercise 8) - 2 rounds, 30 seconds in each direction
- Seated Eagle Arms (Garudasana Arms) (Exercise 9) - 3 rounds, holding each pose for 4 seconds
- Seated Arm Circles (Exercise 10) - 2 rounds, 30 seconds in each direction
- Seated Reverse Prayer Pose (Exercise 11) - 3 rounds, holding each pose for 4 seconds
- Seated Thread the Needle (Exercise 12) - 3 rounds, holding each pose for 4 seconds

Day 23:
- Diaphragmatic Breathing (Exercise 1) - 2 minutes
- Seated Chest Expansion (Exercise 13) - 3 rounds, holding each pose for 4 seconds
- Seated Cow Face Arms (Gomukhasana Arms) (Exercise 14) - 3 rounds, holding each pose for 4 seconds
- Seated Chest Opener (Exercise 15) - 3 rounds, holding each pose for 4 seconds
- Seated Puppy Pose (Exercise 16) - 3 rounds, holding each pose for 4 seconds
- Seated Supported Fish Pose (Exercise 17) - 3 rounds, holding each pose for 4 seconds

Day 24:
- Alternate Nostril Breathing (Nadi Shodhana) (Exercise 2) - 2 minutes
- Seated Forward Bend with Legs Extended (Exercise 18) - 3 rounds, holding each pose for 4 seconds
- Seated Pigeon Pose (Exercise 19) - 3 rounds, holding each pose for 4 seconds
- Seated Tree Pose (Exercise 20) - 3 rounds, holding each pose for 4 seconds
- Seated Hamstring Stretch (Exercise 21) - 3 rounds, holding each pose for 4 seconds
- Hero's Pose (Exercise 22) - 3 rounds, holding each pose for 4 seconds

Day 25:
- Diaphragmatic Breathing (Exercise 1) - 2 minutes
- Seated Foot and Ankle Rolls (Exercise 23) - 2 rounds, 30 seconds in each direction
- Seated Leg Lifts (Exercise 24) - 3 rounds, holding each pose for 4 seconds
- Seated Knee to Chest (Exercise 25) - 3 rounds, holding each pose for 4 seconds
- Seated Calf Raises (Exercise 26) - 3 rounds, holding each pose for 4 seconds
- Seated Toe Taps (Exercise 27) - 2 rounds, 30 seconds each round

Day 26:
- Alternate Nostril Breathing (Nadi Shodhana) (Exercise 2) - 2 minutes
- Seated Leg Extensions (Exercise 28) - 3 rounds, holding each pose for 4 seconds
- Seated Leg Circles (Exercise 29) - 2 rounds, 30 seconds in each direction
- Chair Yoga Lunge Pose (Exercise 30) - 3 rounds, holding each pose for 4 seconds
- Half Supine Pose (Exercise 31) - 3 rounds, holding each pose for 4 seconds
- Seated Eagle Legs (Exercise 32) - 3 rounds, holding each pose for 4 seconds

Day 27:
- Diaphragmatic Breathing (Exercise 1) - 2 minutes
- Side Angle Pose (Exercise 33) - 3 rounds, holding each pose for 4 seconds
- Child's Pose (Exercise 34) - 3 rounds, holding each pose for 4 seconds
- Seated Figure-4 Stretch (Exercise 35) - 3 rounds, holding each pose for 4 seconds
- Seated Butterfly Pose (Exercise 36) - 3 rounds, holding each pose for 4 seconds

Day 28:
- Alternate Nostril Breathing (Nadi Shodhana) (Exercise 2) - 2 minutes
- Seated Forward Bend (Exercise 37) - 3 rounds, holding each pose for 4 seconds.
- Seated Triangle Pose (Exercise 38) - 3 rounds, holding each pose for 4 seconds.
- Bow and Arrow Pose (Exercise 39) - 3 rounds, holding each pose for 4 seconds.
- Seated Bound Angle Pose (Exercise 40) - 3 rounds, holding each pose for 4 seconds.

Day 29:
- Diaphragmatic Breathing (Exercise 1) - 2 minutes
- Seated Mountain Pose (Exercise 41) - 3 rounds, holding each pose for 4 seconds.
- Seated Chair Pose (Exercise 42) - 3 rounds, holding each pose for 4 seconds.
- Crescent Moon Bend (Exercise 43) - 3 rounds, holding each pose for 4 seconds.
- Seated Warrior III (Exercise 44) - 3 rounds, holding each pose for 4 seconds.

Day 30:
- Alternate Nostril Breathing (Nadi Shodhana) (Exercise 2) - 2 minutes
- Sun Salutations (Exercise 45) - 3 rounds, holding each pose for 4 seconds.
- Seated Eagle Balance (Exercise 46) - 3 rounds, holding each pose for 4 seconds.
- Seated Half Moon Balance (Exercise 47) - 3 rounds, holding each pose for 4 seconds.
- Seated Boat Pose (Exercise 48) - 3 rounds, holding each pose for 4 seconds.
- Seated Single-Leg Balance (Exercise 49) - 3 rounds, holding each pose for 4 seconds.
- Seated Dancer's Pose (Exercise 50) - 3 rounds, holding each pose for 4 seconds.

Congratulations on completing the 30-day Chair Yoga program! Through dedicated and regular practice of these exercises, you have made a substantial stride towards enhancing your overall health, stability, mobility, and well-being. Always prioritize your well-being and avoid overexertion. As you continue your chair yoga journey, you can gradually increase the number of rounds and the duration of holding each pose to further enhance your progress.

CHAPTER 13
MEDITATION: A THERAPY AT HOME

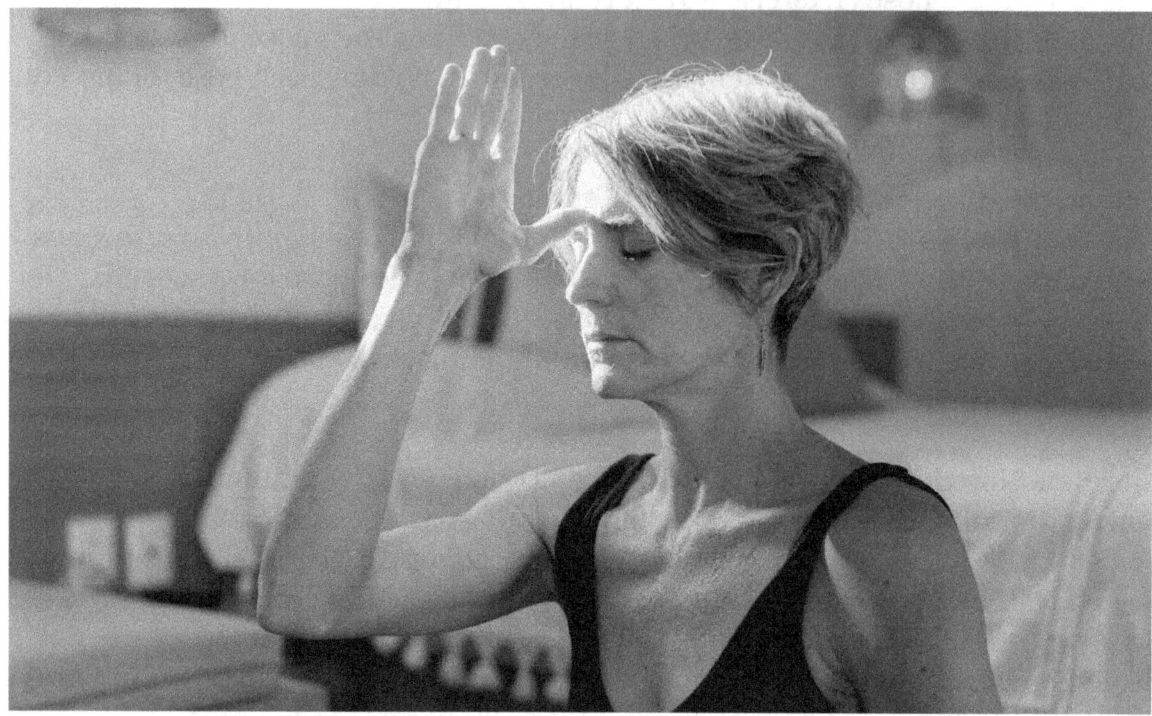

Meditation is a technique for honing the mind's ability to concentrate and steer thoughts. It is commonly employed to enhance awareness, diminish stress, and foster relaxation. Although meditation originated within various religious and spiritual traditions, it has gained widespread popularity in non-religious settings as a method for improving general well-being.

The essence of meditation lies in developing mindfulness, which involves being completely present and involved in the moment without passing judgment. It entails observing one's thoughts, emotions, physical sensations, and the environment around with an open and curious attitude.

Mindfulness meditation is one of the predominant forms of meditation practiced today. In mindfulness meditation, practitioners typically sit quietly and focus on their breath or a particular sensation in the body. When thoughts arise, they're acknowledged without judgment and gently brought back to the focal point, such as the breath. This approach fosters a state of non-reactive mindfulness, focusing purely on the present.

Loving-kindness meditation is another widely embraced method. In this practice, practitioners nurture feelings of love, compassion, and goodwill toward themselves and others. Often, they quietly recite affirmations like "May I be happy, may I be healthy, may I be safe, may I live with ease," directing these benevolent wishes first to themselves and then progressively to loved ones, acquaintances, and even those they may struggle with. This helps expand the circle of compassion outward, promoting a sense of universal kindness.

Other types of meditation include body scan meditation, where attention is systematically directed to different parts of the body, and visualization meditation, where practitioners imagine themselves in a peaceful or serene setting.

Regardless of the specific technique used, the underlying principles of meditation remain the same. It's about training the mind to become more aware of the present moment, cultivating a sense of inner peace, and developing greater clarity and insight into one's thoughts and emotions.

Regular meditation practice has been extensively researched and shown to offer a wide array of benefits for both mental and physical health. For instance, numerous studies indicate that meditation can alleviate symptoms associated with anxiety, depression, and stress. It also enhances focus, concentration, and overall cognitive abilities.

On a physiological level, meditation contributes to changes in the brain that aid in better mood regulation, emotional processing, and resilience to stress. Neuroimaging studies, for example, have demonstrated that meditation can increase the thickness of brain regions involved in managing attention and processing sensory information.

Moreover, meditation positively affects the body's response to stress. It can reduce cortisol levels, which are typically elevated during stress, and decrease inflammation, a factor often linked to various chronic health issues.

Beyond its mental and physical advantages, meditation also offers spiritual benefits for many, enriching their overall sense of well-being. By cultivating a deeper sense of connection with oneself and others, meditation can foster feelings of gratitude, compassion, and interconnectedness.

Despite its numerous benefits, meditation can be challenging for beginners. Many people struggle with distractions, restlessness, or a wandering mind. However, these are all normal experiences, and the key is to approach meditation with patience, kindness, and a non-judgmental attitude.

Importance of Meditative Practices in Daily Lives

Incorporating a meditative practice into everyday life holds profound importance, offering a gateway to deeper self-awareness, enhanced mental clarity, and a more profound connection to the present moment. Beyond the well-documented benefits of stress reduction and anxiety management, meditation serves as a foundational pillar for holistic well-being. Let's delve deeper into why integrating meditative practices into our daily routines is so crucial.

CULTIVATING PRESENCE

It is easy to become lost in the maelstrom of everyday responsibilities, interruptions, and demands in today's fast-paced society. However, when we prioritize meditation, we carve out sacred space to simply be present with ourselves. This deliberate stop enables us to disengage from the continual flow of ideas and really embrace the abundance of the here and now. By training ourselves to be in the here and now via meditation, we may connect with ourselves, others, and the world more profoundly and enjoy life to the fullest.

FOSTERING GRATITUDE

It is easy to lose sight of the little pleasures and gifts in the middle of the fast-paced modern world. Meditation provides a sanctuary for cultivating gratitude, inviting us to slow down and savor the beauty and abundance that surrounds us. By shifting our focus from what's lacking to what's already present, meditation helps us cultivate a mindset of abundance and appreciation. Through regular practice, we begin to recognize and acknowledge the countless blessings that enrich our lives, fostering a profound sense of contentment and fulfillment.

Creativity flourishes in the fertile soil of a quiet mind. When we engage in meditative practices, we create space for inspiration to flow freely, unencumbered by the noise of mental chatter. Meditation encourages us to tap into the wellspring of our inner wisdom, unlocking fresh insights, perspectives, and ideas. Whether through focused concentration or open awareness, meditation provides a fertile ground for creative expression to blossom. By regularly nurturing our creative spirit through meditation, we cultivate a sense of playfulness, curiosity, and innovation that infuses every aspect of our lives.

CULTIVATING COMPASSION

In a world fraught with division, polarization, and conflict, cultivating compassion is more important than ever. Meditation is a powerful means of cultivating compassion, not just towards ourselves but also towards others. Through methods like loving-kindness meditation, we actively send wishes of well-being, happiness, and peace to ourselves, our loved ones, people we know, and even those we might find challenging. This practice helps broaden our empathy and understanding, strengthening our emotional connections with others. By fostering an attitude of kindness, empathy, and understanding, meditation helps dissolve the barriers that separate us, fostering a sense of interconnectedness and unity.

DEEPENING SELF-REFLECTION

Self-reflection is a cornerstone of personal growth and development. Meditation provides a sacred space for deep introspection, inviting us to explore the landscape of our inner world with honesty and compassion. Mindfulness meditation and body scan meditation are techniques that help us become more aware of ourselves and our thoughts and feelings. We may learn a lot about the habits, patterns, and beliefs that impact our life by watching our thoughts, feelings, and bodily sensations with an open mind and an attitude of nonjudgment. Being more self-aware allows us to live our lives in accordance with our beliefs and goals, which in turn strengthens our feeling of honesty and morality.

Cultivating Resilience:

Life is full of challenges, setbacks, and uncertainties. Meditation serves as a powerful tool for cultivating resilience in the face of adversity. By training the mind to remain calm and centered amidst the storms of life, meditation helps us navigate challenges with grace and equanimity. Developing the ability to perceive challenging emotions and sensations without being overwhelmed by them is a goal of mindfulness meditation and breath awareness techniques. Because of this inner strength, we are able to overcome obstacles, adjust to new circumstances, and recover quickly from failures.

Incorporating a meditative practice into everyday life is not merely a luxury but a necessity for navigating the complexities of modern existence with grace, wisdom, and resilience. By cultivating presence, fostering gratitude, enhancing creativity, nurturing compassion, deepening self-reflection, and cultivating resilience, meditation empowers us to live more fully, authentically, and joyfully. As we embark on this journey of self-discovery and transformation, may we embrace the transformative power of meditation as a guiding light illuminating the path to greater peace, purpose, and fulfillment.

There are several tips that can help make meditation more accessible and enjoyable:

1. **The first piece of advice is to take it easy at first. If you've never meditated before, try meditating for only a few minutes a day.**
2. Find a comfortable position: Whether you like to sit, lie down, or stand, pick a posture

that you can maintain comfortably during your meditation session.

3. **Focus on the breath:** The breath is a common focal point in meditation because it's always accessible and can help anchor your awareness in the present moment.

4. **Be kind to yourself: While meditation, the mind naturally wanders. If you find that your mind wanders, just be aware of it and bring it back to the breath or your selected place of concentration.**

5. **Keep at it:** The secret to successful meditation is frequent practice. Every day, even if it's only for a little while, make sure you practice.

6. **Try out many approaches:** You shouldn't be scared to try out a few various types of meditation until you discover the one that suits you best.

As a whole, meditation is a very effective and easy way to improve your health. A higher quality of life, less stress, and clearer thinking are all possible outcomes of regular practice of mindfulness and awareness. Anyone may reap the everyday advantages of meditation with practice, determination, and an open mind.

Addressing Fears and Anxieties Through Breathwork

While meditation offers a general approach to managing anxiety, specific breathing techniques can be particularly helpful in addressing fears and anxieties. Here's how breathwork can be a powerful tool:

- **The Connection Between Breath and Anxiety:** Anxiety or fear triggers our body's fight-or-flight response, characterized by shallow and rapid breathing. This pattern of breathing can escalate the anxiety we feel.
- **The Benefits of Deep Breathing:** Engaging in deep, slow breaths can stimulate the body's relaxation response. This directly opposes the fight-or-flight response by decreasing the heart rate, reducing blood pressure, and fostering a sense of calm.
- **Breathwork Techniques for Anxiety Management:**
  - **Diaphragmatic Breathing (Belly Breathing):** This method requires deep breathing from your diaphragm, which is located between your chest and abdomen. During inhalation, your belly should expand, and during exhalation, it should contract. Aim for slow and steady breaths, inhaling for about 4-6 seconds and exhaling for 6-8 seconds.
  - **Alternate Nostril Breathing (Nadi Shodhana):** This technique involves alternating your breathing through each nostril. Sit in a comfortable position with your spine straight. Use your thumb to close your right nostril and inhale slowly through your left nostril. Pause briefly, then use your ring finger to close your left nostril and exhale slowly through your right nostril. Next, inhale through the right nostril, pause, and exhale through the left. Continue this pattern for several minutes.
- **Tips for Effective Breathwork Practice:**
  - Find a serene and cozy spot to settle into. You can close your eyes gently for relaxation or maintain a soft focus on a point ahead of you.
  - Start with brief sessions, gradually increasing their length as you feel more at ease. Begin with 5-minute sessions and aim for 10-15 minutes as you make this a regular habit.

- Pay attention to your breathing. Feel the coolness as you inhale through your nostrils and the warmth as you exhale. Notice how your belly rises and falls with each breath, practicing diaphragmatic breathing.
- It's normal for your mind to wander, so don't feel discouraged. Simply acknowledge the distraction and gently guide your focus back to your breath without any judgment.
- Stay patient and committed to your practice. Over time, integrating breathwork into your routine will prove increasingly effective in managing your fears and anxieties.

Incorporating Breathwork into Meditation

Breathwork can be a powerful complement to your meditation practice. Here's how to integrate it:

- Prior to commencing your meditation session, allocate a few moments to engage in diaphragmatic breathing or alternate nostril breathing. This will assist in creating a sense of tranquility within your mind and body, allowing you to properly prepare for your meditation practice.
- Throughout your meditation practice, you can utilize your breath as a point of reference to maintain your concentration. Focus on the innate rhythm of your breath without attempting to manipulate it. When you find your thoughts drifting, refocus your attention on the feeling of your breath.
- Following your meditation session, allocate a few additional moments to engage in deep, deliberate breathing. This will assist in incorporating the advantages of meditation and further enhancing sensations of relaxation and well-being.

By incorporating breathwork techniques into your meditation practice, you can create a powerful tool for managing fears, anxieties, and promoting overall well-being.

Conclusion

Meditation and breathwork are powerful tools for cultivating inner peace, reducing stress, and managing anxiety. By integrating these practices into your daily routine, you can cultivate a stronger sense of resilience and effectively navigate the challenges that life presents with a sense of ease and poise. Keep in mind that meditation is a continuous process, rather than a final goal. Take your time, be gentle with yourself, and savor the journey of self-exploration and growth.

Chapter 14
Basic Rules of Nutrition during the Practice Month

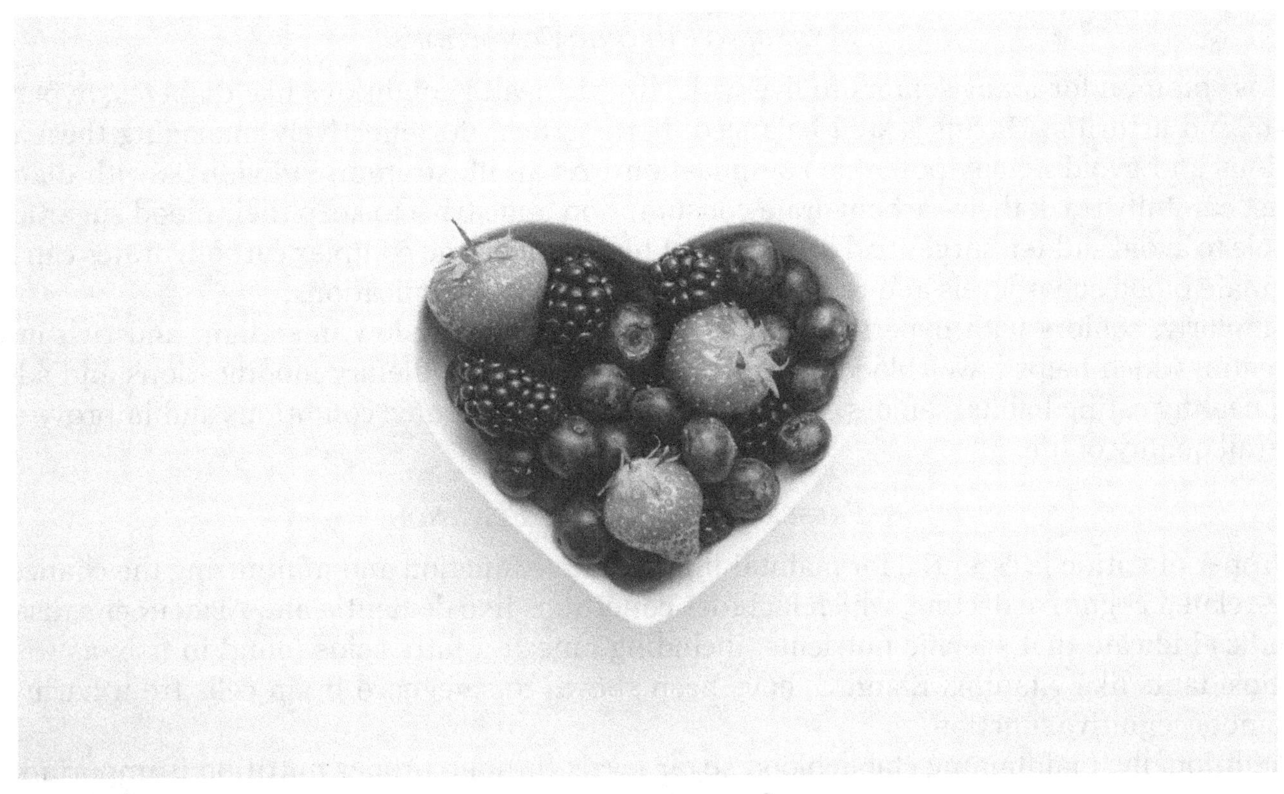

"Let food be thy medicine and medicine be thy food."
- Hippocrates

Nutrition plays a critical role in the overall health and well-being of individuals, regardless of age. However, as people age, their nutritional needs may change, making it especially important for seniors to pay close attention to what they eat. In this essay, we will explore the reasons why nutrition is crucial for seniors, focusing on the various ways it impacts their health and quality of life.

Nutrition: An Essential

Maintaining Physical Health

One of the primary reasons why nutrition is essential for seniors is its impact on physical health. As people get older, their bodies experience changes that can impact their nutrient absorption and overall functioning. Maintaining a balanced diet that includes all the necessary nutrients like vitamins, minerals, proteins, and fiber is essential for supporting overall bodily functions and preventing the development of different health issues.

As an illustration, maintaining bone health and lowering the risk of osteoporosis requires a sufficient intake of calcium and vitamin D. Osteoporosis is a condition where bones become weakened and more susceptible to fractures. In the same way, incorporating foods that are rich in antioxidants, like fruits and vegetables, into your diet can provide protection against age-related illnesses like cancer and cardiovascular disease.

In addition, nutrition is crucial for maintaining a strong immune system, especially as people get older and become more vulnerable to infections and illnesses. A diet rich in nutrients helps strengthen the immune response, reducing the risk of infections and promoting faster recovery from illness.

MANAGING CHRONIC CONDITIONS

It is common for many seniors to live with chronic health conditions like diabetes, hypertension, and arthritis. Having a well-balanced diet is crucial for effectively managing these conditions and avoiding any potential complications. As an illustration, individuals with diabetes must carefully track their carbohydrate consumption and strive to keep their blood sugar levels stable to avoid sudden surges and drops. A diet high in fiber and complex carbohydrates can help regulate blood sugar levels and reduce the risk of diabetic complications.

Similarly, seniors with hypertension can benefit from a diet low in sodium and rich in potassium, which helps lower blood pressure levels. By making dietary modifications and adopting healthy eating habits, seniors can better manage their chronic conditions and improve their overall quality of life.

PRESERVING COGNITIVE FUNCTION

Proper nutrition is essential for maintaining cognitive function and minimizing the chances of age-related cognitive decline, which includes conditions like dementia and Alzheimer's disease. Studies indicate that specific nutrients, including omega-3 fatty acids found in fish, as well as antioxidants like vitamins E and C, have been shown to safeguard brain cells from harm and promote cognitive function.

Additionally, maintaining stable blood sugar levels through proper nutrition is important for preventing cognitive impairment, as fluctuations in blood sugar levels can negatively impact brain function. Consuming a diet rich in fruits, vegetables, whole grains, and healthy fats can provide the nutrients necessary for optimal brain health and cognitive function in seniors.

ENHANCING ENERGY LEVELS AND VITALITY

Proper nutrition is essential for seniors to maintain their energy levels and stay engaged in their daily activities. As individuals age, they may experience a decline in energy levels and muscle mass, making it essential to consume nutrient-dense foods that provide sustained energy and support muscle health.

A diet rich in lean proteins, complex carbohydrates, and healthy fats can help seniors maintain muscle mass, strength, and endurance, allowing them to participate in activities they enjoy and maintain their independence. Additionally, staying hydrated by drinking an adequate amount of water is crucial for supporting energy levels and preventing dehydration, which can exacerbate fatigue and contribute to other health issues.

IMPROVING DIGESTIVE HEALTH

Digestive issues are common among seniors, including constipation, indigestion, and gastrointestinal discomfort. Unhealthy dietary habits, like consuming processed foods that are high in fat and sugar, can worsen these problems and have a negative effect on digestive health. Nevertheless, seniors can enhance their digestive health and regularity by adopting a well-rounded diet that incorporates ample fiber-rich foods like fruits, vegetables, whole grains, and legumes.

Fiber plays a crucial role in maintaining bowel regularity and preventing constipation. It achieves this by increasing the volume of the stool and aiding its smooth passage through the digestive system. In addition, incorporating probiotic-rich foods like yogurt and kefir into your diet can support a healthy balance of gut bacteria, which is crucial for optimal digestion and a strong immune system.

Promoting Emotional Well-being

Ultimately, nutrition is crucial for fostering emotional well-being and mental health in older adults. Adopting a nutritious diet can greatly enhance mood and cognitive function, lowering the likelihood of experiencing depression and anxiety. On the other hand, seniors who have unhealthy eating habits and lack essential nutrients are more likely to experience mental health disorders.

Consuming foods rich in omega-3 fatty acids, such as salmon, walnuts, and flaxseeds, has been shown to have antidepressant effects and improve overall mood and well-being. Additionally, maintaining stable blood sugar levels through balanced nutrition can help prevent mood swings and promote emotional stability.

In conclusion, nutrition is of utmost importance for seniors, as it plays a vital role in maintaining physical health, managing chronic conditions, preserving cognitive function, enhancing energy levels, improving digestive health, and promoting emotional well-being. By adopting healthy eating habits and consuming a well-balanced diet rich in essential nutrients, seniors can improve their quality of life and enjoy a happier, healthier, and more active retirement. It's always a good idea to focus on nutrition and make beneficial adjustments to promote overall health and well-being as you age.

Basic Rules for a Nutritious Diet

- **Maintain Hydration:** It's important for seniors to stay hydrated by drinking water regularly, including before, during, and after yoga sessions, to keep the body functioning optimally.
- **Emphasize Whole Foods:** Prioritize nutrient-rich whole foods like fruits, vegetables, whole grains, lean proteins, and healthy fats for their essential nutrients, antioxidants, and fiber, supporting overall health.
- **Achieve Balance in Meals:** Strive for balanced meals with a mix of carbohydrates, protein, and healthy fats to provide energy, support muscle repair, and promote satiety and nutrient absorption.
- **Practice Mindful Eating:** Be mindful of hunger and fullness cues, eat slowly, and savor each bite to prevent overeating and aid digestion.
- **Limit Processed Foods and Sugars:** Reduce consumption of processed foods and snacks high in added sugars, as they offer little nutritional value and can lead to energy fluctuations and inflammation.
- **Incorporate Anti-Inflammatory Foods:** Include foods like berries, fatty fish, nuts, seeds, olive oil, and turmeric to help reduce inflammation and support overall health, especially for conditions like arthritis.
- **Listen to Your Body:** Pay attention to how different foods affect your body and choose those that leave you feeling energized and nourished.
- **Pre- and Post-Workout Nutrition:** Before yoga, opt for light snacks such as fruit or yogurt for energy without feeling too full. Afterward, have a balanced meal with protein,

carbohydrates, and healthy fats to aid muscle recovery and replenish energy.
- **Be Consistent:** Consistently follow a balanced and nutritious diet to support both your yoga practice and overall well-being.
- **Consult a Dietitian:** Seek personalized nutrition advice from a registered dietitian if you have specific dietary concerns or health conditions. They can offer tailored guidance to meet your individual needs and goals.

By following these basic rules of nutrition, seniors can support their yoga practice and promote overall health and vitality during the practice month.

CONCLUSION

As we conclude our exploration of chair yoga for seniors, it is important to recognize that this transformative practice is just one piece of the puzzle when it comes to achieving optimal health and well-being in our golden years. While chair yoga offers a wealth of benefits, from improved flexibility and strength to enhanced mental clarity and emotional balance, it is essential to approach wellness from a holistic perspective.

Incorporating Other Light Sports and Physical Activities

In addition to a consistent chair yoga practice, seniors can benefit greatly from engaging in other light sports and physical activities. These complementary practices can help further improve overall fitness, prevent boredom, and provide a well-rounded approach to maintaining an active lifestyle. Some excellent options to consider include:

- Wall Pilates: This low-impact, beginner-friendly form of Pilates utilizes the support of a wall to help seniors build core strength, improve posture, and enhance balance. Wall Pilates exercises can be easily adapted to suit individual needs and abilities, making it an accessible and effective choice for older adults.
- Tai Chi: Known for its gentle, flowing movements and meditative qualities, Tai Chi is an ancient Chinese practice that promotes balance, flexibility, and stress reduction. Many senior centers and community organizations offer Tai Chi classes specifically designed for older adults, providing a supportive and social environment for practice.
- Walking: One of the simplest and most accessible forms of exercise, walking offers numerous health benefits for seniors, including improved cardiovascular health, increased bone density, and better mood. You can greatly improve your health by making walking a regular part of your routine, whether it's a brisk neighborhood stroll or a leisurely park promenade.
- Swimming: For seniors with access to a pool, swimming provides an excellent low-impact, full-body workout. For people who suffer from arthritis, back pain, or any number of other physical restrictions, swimming is a great option because of the buoyancy that helps them avoid strain on their muscles and joints. Many community pools offer senior-friendly classes, such as aqua aerobics or water walking, providing a fun and social way to stay active.

Throughout this book, we have emphasized the importance of consistency in your chair yoga practice. Dedicating just 15 minutes a day to your practice can yield significant improvements in physical, mental, and emotional well-being over time. Remember, the key to success is not the length of your practice, but the regularity with which you engage in it.

For optimal consistency, it is recommended to establish a dedicated time slot for your chair yoga practice every day. This could be in the morning as soon as you wake up or right before you go to sleep. Create a designated space in your home that feels peaceful and inviting, and keep any necessary props, such as a sturdy chair or yoga blocks, easily accessible. By making your practice a non-negotiable part of your daily routine, you will be more likely to stick with it and reap the numerous benefits it offers.

In addition to the physical benefits of chair yoga, this practice also offers a powerful tool for addressing fears, anxieties, and other emotional challenges that may arise in our senior years. By practicing mindful breathing, meditation, and focusing on the present moment, chair yoga offers seniors the opportunity to enhance their inner peace, resilience, and emotional balance.

When facing fears or anxieties, it is important to remember the significance of focusing on your breath. Take a moment to relax and center yourself by taking a few slow, deep breaths. Pay attention to the gentle flow of air as it enters and leaves your body. This straightforward practice of focused breathing can assist in soothing the nervous system, stilling the mind, and restoring a sense of balance.

The Ripple Effect: Inspiring Others and Building Community

As you continue on your chair yoga journey, you may find that your practice not only transforms your own life but also inspires those around you. By sharing your experiences and enthusiasm with friends, family, and fellow seniors, you can help spread the message of the life-changing power of chair yoga and encourage others to give it a try.

Consider inviting a friend to join you for a chair yoga session, or share your favorite resources, such as this book or online videos, with those who may be interested in starting their own practice. You might even consider organizing a small chair yoga group within your community, creating a supportive and social environment for seniors to come together and prioritize their health and well-being.

Remember, the impact of your practice extends far beyond the confines of your yoga mat or chair. By embracing the transformative power of chair yoga and sharing it with others, you have the potential to create a ripple effect of positive change, fostering a greater sense of connection, compassion, and vitality within your community.

A Final Word of Encouragement

As we come to the end of this journey, we want to leave you with a final word of encouragement. Starting a chair yoga practice requires a strong commitment, determination, and a readiness to push your boundaries. There may be times when you feel challenged, frustrated, or uncertain, but remember that these moments are all part of the process of growth and self-discovery.

Trust in the wisdom of your body, and approach your practice with patience, compassion, and a spirit of curiosity. Acknowledge your achievements, regardless of their size, and view any obstacles as chances to gain knowledge and adapt your strategy.

Above all, remember that you are worthy of the time, energy, and effort you invest in your own well-being. By prioritizing your health and happiness through the practice of chair yoga, you are not only improving your own quality of life but also setting a powerful example for others to follow.

So, as you continue on this path of self-care and self-discovery, know that you are supported, valued, and capable of achieving extraordinary things. May your chair yoga practice be a source of joy, strength, and inner peace, and may it help you navigate the challenges and triumphs of your senior years with grace, resilience, and an open heart.